LIVING WITH HEPATITIS C

A Survivor's Guide

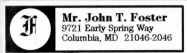

A SELF-HELP CLASSIC™

HATHERLEIGH PRESS

Hatherleigh Press
1114 First Avenue, Suite 500
New York, NY 10021
1-800-906-1234

DISCLAIMER
This book does not give legal or medical advice.
Always consult your lawyer, doctor, and other professionals.
The names of people who contributed anecdotal material have been changed.

The ideas and suggestions contained in this book are not intended as a substitute
for consulting with a physician. All matters regarding your health require medical
supervision.

Library of Congress Cataloging-in-Publication Data

Everson, Gregory T., 1950–
Living with hepatitis C : a survivor's guide / by Gregory T. Everson
and Hedy Weinberg.
    p. cm.
  Includes bibliographical references and index.
  ISBN 1–57826–003–5 (pbk. : alk. paper)
    1. Hepatitis C—Popular works.   I. Weinberg, Hedy, 1939–
II. Title.
RC848.H425E95 1997
362. 1'963623—dc21   97–29792
                                              CIP

All Hatherleigh Press titles are available for special promotions and premiums.
For more information, please contact the manager of our Special Sales department.

Designed by Dede Cummings Designs
Printed in Canada on acid-free paper ∞
10 9 8 7 6 5 4 3 2 1

DEDICATION

I wish to thank my family for tolerating my "late hours" of work, absence from home, and long periods at the computer. My wife, Linda, is an artist whose creativity has inspired me to exercise my own minuscule creative talents. My sons, Brad and Todd, represent my heart and soul and I am extremely proud of who they are, what they have done, and I anxiously await their future accomplishments. Finally, I must acknowledge my father, Lloyd K. Everson, and mother, Ruth Everson, whose support, both personal and financial, was a constant source of strength that was greatly appreciated. To all my family, friends, and colleagues I thank you and hope you get a chance to read this work. Let me know if it is worthy of your readership.

Gregory T. Everson, M.D.

To my husband, Michael, my love, a truly good person who stands up for what's right, yet keeps a sense of humor, warmth, and openness. Your support, encouragement, and belief in this book made its creation possible. And to our children Ben, Adam, Shira and David, who offered help and cheered me on—I'm proud of you, your values, and your strong sense of family.

Hedy Weinberg

In memory of Fred Kern, Jr., M.D., the authors and the publisher will contribute a portion of the profits from this book to the Kern Research Foundation for the Understanding and Treatment of Gastrointestinal and Liver Diseases to further hepatitis C research.

Kern Foundation
7500 East Dartmouth Avenue, No. 30
Denver, Colorado 80231-4264
Telephone (303) 750-5509
Facsimile (303) 750-4688

CONTENTS

PREFACE

*L*iving with Hepatitis C: A Survivor's Guide grew out of a need I saw at the University of Colorado Health Sciences Center. When the first test for the virus became available around 1990, newly diagnosed patients asked questions but, unfortunately, we physicians had relatively few answers. As the years went by, our knowledge grew, and so did the task of educating the rapidly growing number of people diagnosed with hepatitis C.

To meet the public's need for information about hepatitis C, I began to give lectures specifically targeted to patients and their families. After one lecture, Hedy Weinberg, a hepatitis C patient and writer, approached me and suggested that we turn the lecture series into a guidebook for our patients at the clinic. What began as a simple pamphlet quickly turned into a long-term project. In these pages you will hear the voices of patients and staff at the University Hospital and the University of Colorado Health Sciences Center who generously contributed their knowledge and experiences and encouraged us to complete the work.

As we wrote and rewrote the text, we tried to create a useful guide that would take the patient step-by-step through the process of diagnosis and ongoing care. We tried to anticipate questions, translate medical jargon, and reduce the fear of the unknown. Therefore, we also presented overviews of emotional, financial, and nutritional issues that accompany this chronic illness.

Our goal was to help people cope with a disease that affects almost four million Americans. In a short clinical visit, people often keep a "stiff upper lip." But for this book, patients shared their experiences—the funny and hopeful times, as well as the frightening, sad moments. I gained a new appreciation and insight into my patients' lives.

Throughout the book we emphasize the need for thoughtful well-controlled clinical and basic research of hepatitis C. The final chapter speculates on potential breakthroughs in virology, cell biology, and medicine that might lead to a cure of this disease. My own career has been centered around investigation and research. I owe much of my interest to my recently deceased mentor, colleague, and friend, Dr. Fred Kern, Jr. The Kern Foundation was established in Dr. Kern's name to foster research into the causes and cures of gastrointestinal and liver disease. Both Hedy and I, as well as Hatherleigh Press, will contribute a percentage of the proceeds from the sale of this book to the Kern Foundation for the express purpose of advancing research into hepatitis C.

One last word: Although *Living with Hepatitis C: A Survivor's Guide* is a detailed reference guide, it does not replace the advice and care of your physician, nor does it give legal advice. Instead, it is designed solely to educate patients and their families about hepatitis C and how it affects their lives. Consult appropriate specialists and always work closely with your doctor when making medical decisions.

ACKNOWLEDGMENTS

With appreciation and gratitude to the hard-working, dedicated members of the Section of Hepatology, University of Colorado Health Sciences Center—and with special thanks to Michelle Eto, who supported and helped us every step of the way: Bahri Bilir, M.D.; Thomas Trouillot, M.D.; Roshan Shrestha, M.D.; Igal Kam, M.D., Chief of Division of Transplant Surgery, University of Colorado Health Sciences Center; Michael Wachs, M.D.; University Hospital anesthesiologists Susan Mandell, M.D., and Jeremy Katz, M.D.; Robert House, M.D., Director of Residency Training and the Department of Psychiatric Consultation Liaison Service; Thomas Beresford, M.D.; Barbara Fey, R.N., M.S.N., Hepatology Nurse; Cathy Ray, R.N., B.S.N., M.A., Hepatology Nurse; Nancy Barfield, R.N., Hepatology Nurse; Justin Skilbred, M.A., Hepatology Assistant; Claire Reilly, R.N., Research Coordinator; Tracy Mulcahy, R.N., B.S.N., Research Coordinator; Carol McKinley, R.N., Research Coordinator; Radene Showalter, Laboratory Researcher; Tracy Steinberg, R.N., M.S., C.C.T.C.; Cathy Morgan, R.N.; Michael Talamantes, M.S.S.W., L.C.S.W.; Katherine (Katy) L. Paulson, R.D., Adult Renal/Transplant Dietician; Chip Webb, M.S.H.A., M.B.A., Coordinator, Transplant Financial Services; Patty Polsky, M.B.A., Manager, Registration and Financial Services; Rev. Julie Swaney, University Hospital Chaplain; The Children's Hospital, Denver, Colorado, and the Pediatric Transplant Team, including Fritz

Karrer, M.D.; Ronald Sokol, M.D.; and Michael Narkewicz, M.D.

Dr. Everson wishes to further acknowledge the support of the staff at University Hospital and the University of Colorado Health Sciences Center in the care and management of patients with hepatitis C.

In addition, we'd like to thank Meredith Pate-Willig, M.S.W., L.C.S.W., and Robert House, M.D., who gave generously of their time and experience regarding emotional issues of chronic illness; Chip Webb, Coordinator, Transplant Financial Services, who contributed his considerable financial expertise; Denver attorney Gregory W. Heron of Fogel, Keating and Wagner, for his help with our chapter on disability procedures; and hepatology nurses Barbara Fey and Cathy Ray for their comments and suggestions.

Special thanks to The Hep C Connection, especially Ann Jesse, Director; Denise Carter, Betsy Hoover, and support group members; University Hospital's Transplant Support Group; the Rocky Mountain Chapter of the American Liver Foundation, Lee Gerstner, President; and all the hepatitis C patients across the country who shared their stories and touched our lives.

1

What Is Hepatitis C?

An Introduction

I work for a city agency, and we're required to take annual phys-
icals. This year the doctor asked me to come back for more blood
tests. My liver counts were high, he said. That's how I found out
I had hepatitis C.

I'm managing. What else can I do? But my wife—she's
having a tough time. It's hard to believe, but I had never even
heard of hepatitis C before.

Barry

IF YOU'VE JUST BEEN DIAGNOSED with hepati-
tis C, you have a lot of questions: "What is hepatitis C? How
did I acquire the infection? Is there treatment? If I tell them at
work, will they fire me?"

Hepatitis C is a viral infection that causes inflammation, injury, and ultimately scarring of the liver. That sounds frightening,
but try not to panic. You're not alone. Current estimates indicate
that 3.9 million people living in the United States have hepatitis
C. Although hepatitis C is a serious problem, the infection usually
progresses slowly over years or decades. You have time to consider your options.

Take a look at the bottom line. Hepatitis C can be dangerous if it damages your liver to the point of cirrhosis. In fact, 8,000 to 10,000 Americans die each year from liver failure due to hepatitis C—about one in every 400 to 500 patients.

As you can see from the mortality figures, it's far more likely that you will have to learn to *live* with the virus until scientists find a cure. That's what this book is about: how to live with and survive hepatitis C.

By now, you know it's hard to find a lot of information about hepatitis C because it's a newly discovered disease. Researchers didn't develop a screening test until 1990—long after the hepatitis C virus had infected millions of people. Before this time, it was impossible to detect hepatitis C in donated blood. As a result, the nation's blood supply became contaminated.

That's what happened to Hedy Weinberg, who's writing this book with me. She was exposed to hepatitis C through an emergency transfusion. Let me introduce you to Hedy, who will tell you her story—a story you'll hear throughout the book, because it's typical of what most people face:

> *In 1967, I gave birth to a stillborn baby girl. My uterus ruptured, I almost died, and they gave me five pints of plasma. Twenty-six years later, I found out I had hepatitis C. Looking back, it explains some symptoms I've had over the years: a thyroid condition, a slight blood clotting problem, some depression, and fatigue. The transfusion saved my life—but it gave me hepatitis C.*

A Word of Caution: Information in this book does not substitute for the advice of your physician. If you have hepatitis C, you should be under a doctor's care.

In this chapter we'll discuss some basic facts and statistics about hepatitis C, its history and discovery, and information about viruses and other forms of viral hepatitis. Here are the topics we'll cover:

- You Are Not Alone
- A Silent Epidemic

You Are Not Alone

If you, or someone you love, has hepatitis C, know that you're not alone. The U.S. Centers for Disease Control and Prevention (CDC) estimate that 3.9 million Americans are infected. Hepatitis

FIGURE I. WORLDWIDE DISTRIBUTION OF HEPATITIS C

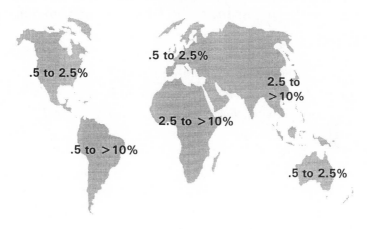

LEGEND: The percentage of patients infected with hepatitis C on each continent is shown. The data for this figure was extracted from the Weekly Epidemiological Record of the World Health Organization (1997).

C is a global problem. The World Health Organization estimates that hepatitis C infects 8.9 million people in Europe and more than 170 million chronic carriers worldwide (see Figure 1).

It's hard to relate to numbers this big, so let's make the statistics more real. The number of people in the United States with hepatitis C is *double* that of HIV/AIDS or Parkinson's and more than *ten* times the number of Americans with multiple sclerosis.

In my state of Colorado, which is quite typical, about 20,000 to 40,000 people have hepatitis C; that's roughly three out of every 350 residents. Although the public doesn't realize it, chronic hepatitis C is the most commonly reported infectious disease in the state.

But numbers and statistics don't tell the whole story. When you're diagnosed with hepatitis C, all of a sudden, you feel as alone as you can possibly feel. It's as if an invisible fence has gone up between you and all the other people who don't have hepatitis C. You have an infectious illness; they don't. You're worried about yourself, and you're worried about the people you love. You're angry. Perhaps you even feel ashamed.

Hepatitis puts a heavy strain on relationships. Mothers and fathers hesitate to cook for their families. Friends who used to hug and kiss you pull away. People don't tell their bosses and co-workers because they might lose their jobs. Lovers are afraid to touch one another.

> *My wife moved into the other bedroom. The doctor explained that it's okay for us to have sex—that if we're married and we're not sleeping around, there's almost zero risk that she'll get infected.*
>
> *But I don't know. It's like she hears the word "virus," and she freaks out. When I try to hug her, I feel her tense up. It hurts.*
>
> *Tony*

A healthy dose of facts about hepatitis C helps people deal with their fears. You can touch people; you can cook for them. Tell your family, friends, neighbors, and bosses that to get infected, they'd have to have their skin punctured with contaminated blood. Hepatitis C is a blood-to-blood virus. People get it from transfusions, shared drug needles, tattoos, body-piercing, borrowed razors, and so on.

Medical professionals and patients such as hemophiliacs and people on dialysis are at risk because of their exposure to blood and blood products. They make up about 10 percent of the hepatitis C population. Patients with a prior history of blood transfusion account for 20 percent (now, of course, tests screen donated blood for hepatitis C, and the risk of getting hepatitis C from a transfusion is exceedingly low); intravenous drug users represent 20 to 30 percent of cases; and a surprisingly large figure of 40 percent don't know how they came into contact with contaminated blood.

A Silent Epidemic

Hepatitis C is called the silent epidemic because you can have the virus and not know it. It's unusual to have severe symptoms until the end-stages of liver disease—a process that, if it occurs, may take decades. So it's hard for people to believe they're infected. Here's Hedy:

> In December of 1992, I went to my family doctor for a regular checkup. I didn't feel sick, just tired, but that's not unusual for me because I have a thyroid condition. Blood tests showed my liver enzymes were a little above normal. I agreed to stay off alcohol and repeat the tests every month for three months. No change. A specialist ordered more tests and a liver biopsy.
>
> My family doctor called with the results: "Inactive hepatitis C—the best outcome we could hope for." The next day, he phoned again. "There's been a mistake," he said in a sad, tentative voice. "The pathologist reread your slide, and it's mild chronic active hepatitis C."
>
> My stomach clenched. I felt a cold rush of fear, even though I didn't know what hepatitis C was or what to expect.

Hepatitis C usually progresses slowly, with peaks and valleys of activity. Although it's a serious illness, it's important to keep perspective. We now believe that hepatitis C becomes chronic in 85 percent of infected people.

While it's true that one-third of them will develop cirrhosis (scarring of the liver), two-thirds may not. One of five people with cirrhosis may also get hepatocellular carcinoma, a form of liver cancer, but four out of five will not. The frustrating problem is that we can't predict outcomes for individual patients. Interferon treatments boost the immune system but clear the virus in only 10 to 20 percent of cases.

A time bomb, the virus can lurk in the body for decades, silently injuring your liver and setting the stage for complications from liver disease.

> I had a high-detail, difficult job managing a department store, so at first I thought it was too much stress. I felt foggy, confused. I forgot appointments, couldn't concentrate on the paperwork. Finally, I called a doctor. Maybe I was cracking up. I figured he'd give me an anti-depressant.
>
> Two days before my appointment, my eyes turned yellow, my stomach was out to here, and I itched all over. The diagnosis? Cirrhosis, end-stage liver disease caused by hepatitis C. My life narrowed down to two choices: die or get on a waiting list for a liver transplant.
>
> *Jim*

We need to get the word out that hepatitis C is a major public health problem. Many people have no idea they're carrying the virus, but it's the most prevalent form of chronic hepatitis in the United States, accounting for 20 to 25 percent of all hepatitis cases. When did this silent epidemic begin?

The Discovery of Hepatitis C

In the 1970s, researchers developed blood tests to identify the viruses that cause hepatitis A and B. However, it became apparent that many blood samples, responsible for cases of post-transfusion hepatitis, tested negative for A and B. For lack of a better term, scientists called this virus non-A, non-B hepatitis.

Then, in the 1980s—breakthrough! After many years of work, investigators under the direction of Daniel W. Bradley and Michael Houghton at the CDC and Chiron Corporation finally identified the virus in non-A, non-B infected blood. They used specialized genetic chemistry to identify the virus, and with this discovery, they were able to give it a name: hepatitis C.

In 1990 the first test for the hepatitis C virus (HCV) became commercially available. Routine physical examinations and blood bank screens uncovered an explosion of cases.

In my mail yesterday was a letter from the blood bank. They had refused my blood because it showed up positive for hepatitis C. What a shock! I couldn't believe it. I've never been sick a day in my life. What is hepatitis C?

Tom

Understanding Hepatitis C

To understand hepatitis C, it helps to define three terms:

- hepatitis
- virus
- hepatitis C virus or HCV

What Is Hepatitis? Hepatitis simply means inflammation of the liver. Many injurious agents can cause hepatitis, including alcohol, medications, drugs, toxins, or viruses.

Unfortunately, the public hears so many stories of celebrities who injured their livers with substance abuse that they tend to lump all forms of liver disease together. As anyone with hepatitis C can tell you, it's not uncommon (although extremely unfair) to be labeled an alcoholic, even if you've never taken a drink.

When I finally tell someone I have hepatitis C, the atmosphere changes. I've had people give me this airbrush handshake because they don't want to touch me. Or they'll say, "Isn't that what that baseball star had? Didn't he drink himself to death?" Suddenly, there's this invisible wall.

Sara

During the past 30 years, scientists have discovered hepatitis viruses A through G. Each virus has its own ways of infecting people, but it's hard for the public to see the differences.

It's an awkward moment when you let friends know you have this disease. They don't know what to say, and most of what they know about viruses has to do with AIDS, so you get a lot of weird stares and silences. You can see the stereotypes running through their heads. I'm so tired of explaining that the virus is almost never passed sexually, that it's a blood-to-blood thing.

Bob

What Is a Virus? The name virus evokes fear in people, fear of the unknown, the invisible. Viruses are not visible to the human eye or by standard microscopy; you need an electron microscope to see viruses. Despite their small size, viruses carry genetic material with enough punch to injure our organs and bodies and even cause death.

Viruses are as old as humankind—possibly older. Archeologists have unearthed an Egyptian mummy that bears pockmarks, evidence of the smallpox virus thousands of years ago. Among other diseases, viruses cause polio, mononucleosis, rabies, herpes, yellow fever, influenza, measles, rubella, chickenpox, mumps, the common cold—and new plagues, such as Ebola and AIDS.

"A virus," said Nobel Laureate Sir Peter Medawar, "is a piece of bad news wrapped in protein."[1] And that about sums it up. A virus contains a center of nucleic acid (the viral genes) surrounded by a protein coat.

When a virus's coat attaches to a cell in the body, the virus's genes enter the cell. It orders the cell to stop its own work and to make more viruses instead. In time, the virus multiplies to infect other cells.

Alerted to danger, the body's immune system sends out anti-bodies, special types of proteins, to stick to the invading virus and neutralize it. Viruses, however, are able to change and mutate to evade these antibodies.

Unfortunately, the hepatitis C virus is particularly good at mutating, which makes it difficult for scientists to create a vaccine. It's been hard to hit this moving target.

What Is the Hepatitis C Virus (HCV)? HCV is a single-stranded ribonucleic acid (RNA) virus organized like the RNA of flaviviruses, a family of viruses that produce yellow fever, dengue, and Japanese encephalitis. To complicate the hepatitis C picture even more, at least six distinct genetic strains (or genotypes) of the HCV virus have been identified.

The Hepatitis Viral Alphabet

When you tell someone you have hepatitis C, you usually end up fielding a lot of questions that have to do with other forms of viral hepatitis: "Do you get it from sex? From dirty food?" It helps to know the facts about the hepatitis alphabet—from A to G. Take Hedy's situation:

> For a long time, I didn't talk about hepatitis C except to my husband and kids. When I finally told a couple of good friends, I don't know what I expected—sympathy, horror. I didn't expect my friend to make light of the whole thing. "Maybe you ate in a dirty restaurant," she said. "No big deal. You'll be fine." I explained how hepatitis A spread.
>
> When I told a second friend, she looked so uncomfortable, I knew she thought I had been infected sexually. I finally convinced her that she was thinking of hepatitis B.
>
> Neither one understood, and I felt frustrated and annoyed. I don't know why I was so upset. Before I knew I had hepatitis C, I didn't know what the differences among hepatitis viruses were either. It doesn't make sense, but it took me a long time before I felt ready to talk to a friend again.

As you now know, hepatitis means inflammation of the liver. The most common cause of hepatitis is viral. Hepatitis viruses primarily attack the liver, while other viruses (such as the herpes or mononucleosis viruses) injure the liver as part of a generalized infection.

We know at least seven distinct hepatitis viruses, identified by the letters A through G. Blood tests distinguish and diagnose the different forms, but the public tends to lump them all together.

Hepatitis A. Outbreaks of this virus occur because of poor hygiene—a contaminated water supply or, for example, inadequate hand washing in a day-care facility. Hepatitis A, excreted in feces, is the most common cause of food or water-borne epidemic hepatitis.

People who contract hepatitis A typically develop flu-like symptoms within 10 to 40 days of exposure (the acute stage). They experience low-grade fever, muscle aches, joint aches, headache, malaise, anorexia, and mild abdominal pain. Often, but not always, these symptoms are rapidly followed by jaundice, a yellowing of the whites of the eyes and skin. In the vast majority of cases, the patient recovers completely with lifelong immunity against reinfection.

Hepatitis A never persists after the acute infection, so people don't develop chronic hepatitis, cirrhosis, or liver cancer. Rarely, in approximately one out of 1,000 cases, does the patient have severe acute hepatitis leading to liver failure and urgent need for transplantation.

Hepatitis B. Hepatitis B spreads primarily through blood inoculation: transfusions of blood or blood products, intravenous illicit drug use, hemodialysis, cardiac bypass surgery, or accidental needle-stick. It also spreads readily by sexual contact and can easily be transmitted from mother to infant at delivery.

Ninety to 95 percent of adults infected with hepatitis B clear the infection and maintain lifelong immunity. Rarely, a patient may develop liver failure from severe acute hepatitis B. The remaining 5 to 10 percent do not clear the virus. They become carriers or develop chronic hepatitis and risk progression to cirrhosis or liver cancer.

Untreated newborns who acquire hepatitis B from their mothers will often develop lifelong infection. The good news is that treating the newborn with HBIG (hepatitis B immune globulin) and hepatitis B vaccine immediately after delivery prevents transmission in more than 95 percent of cases.

People with acute hepatitis B have the same symptoms as people with any other form of acute hepatitis. Chronic sufferers may not have symptoms or may complain of chronic fatigue, malaise, poor energy, and episodic jaundice.

The only FDA-approved medical therapy for chronic hepatitis B is interferon-alfa, although new antiviral agents (lamivudine, famciclovir) appear to be effective. Patients who need transplants for severe acute hepatitis seldom, if ever, develop hepatitis B in the transplanted liver. The virus may recur in transplants performed for chronic liver disease, but use of lamivudine and long-term immune globulin therapy after the transplantation reduces that risk.

Hepatitis C. Hepatitis C is transmitted by blood, like hepatitis B. However, unlike hepatitis B, it seems to be poorly transmitted by sexual contact and is infrequently passed from an otherwise healthy mother to her newborn.

> *We've been married 15 years. I told my wife—and the doctor told my wife—that she doesn't have hepatitis C after sleeping with me all these years, and that it would be extremely rare to get it from sex.*
>
> *We could use protection if that would help her feel safer. But it's pretty lonely. She doesn't even hug me anymore.*
>
> *Ralph*

Most infected people may not be aware they have had a past episode of acute hepatitis. In general, symptoms of acute hepatitis C are mild and liver enzyme elevations in the blood are modest. Chronically infected patients may have identical symptoms and liver enzyme tests but very different results from a biopsy—from mild, benign histology (the study of the liver tissue under the microscope) to advanced injury with cirrhosis.

Patients may be candidates for interferon therapy. New agents currently under investigation or development include ribavirin, thymosin, amantadine and protease inhibitors. Twenty to 40 percent of patients on liver transplant waiting lists have hepatitis C.

Hepatitis D. Hepatitis D, or delta hepatitis, is an incomplete virus that requires the presence of hepatitis B in order to complete its life cycle. For this reason, delta is typically found only in patients who have hepatitis B. Risk factors are the same as for hepatitis B. Hepatitis B patients coinfected with delta have a greater chance of developing fulminant hepatitis (a sudden, severe attack), more severe chronic active hepatitis, and an increased rate of progression to cirrhosis. The virus does not seem to have a major effect on hepatitis B patients' response to interferon therapy or on their survival or on the recurrence of hepatitis B after a liver transplant.

Hepatitis E. Symptoms are the same as hepatitis A, but cases in the United States appear to be imports from Central America, Mexico, and the Indian subcontinent of Asia. In most instances, patients don't become chronic carriers, and the virus is not associated with hepatocellular cancer.

Currently no vaccine or specific medical therapy exists. If acquired during pregnancy, hepatitis E has been associated with high rates of maternal and fetal mortality. The Centers for Disease Control in Atlanta, GA, offer testing.

Hepatitis F. The story is not fully in on this virus. Early reports have suggested that it may cause sporadic hepatitis with rare progression to liver failure. Only a few specialized research laboratories can test for this virus.

Hepatitis G. We're learning more about this newly discovered virus, which is transmitted in the same way as hepatitis C. Hepatitis C and hepatitis G are in the same family of viruses, and hepatitis G is comprised of at least four main subtypes. But we don't know whether hepatitis G causes clinically significant liver disease.

Reports indicate that as many as 20 percent of hepatitis C patients may also be infected with hepatitis G. However, there's no evidence that hepatitis G independently causes chronic progressive hepatitis.

Hepatitis C: How Close Is a Cure?

Viruses are so complex, they can be a frustrating experience for patients who want to know more about them. Here's Hedy's experience:

> *I'm a p.k.—a preacher's kid—and I'd always been taught that it was good to study and learn and understand. So when I knew I had hepatitis C, I ran to the library.*
>
> *As a writer, I've done medical research before, but I couldn't make sense out of the numbers and initials and blood types and medical jargon. It was really frustrating. It took awhile for me to relax and admit that it was beyond me. It took even longer to realize that part of the problem was that scientists didn't have the answers either.*

Researchers are beginning to grow the HCV virus in the laboratory to find out how the virus reproduces. Scientists at Chiron Corporation recently were able to cultivate hepatitis C in a continuous liver cell line. If their work, and the work of other laboratories, checks out, this could lead to a better understanding of how the virus gains entry to our liver cells and how it reproduces. This knowledge would be instrumental to developing new drugs and therapy to fight hepatitis C.

Once we know how the virus reproduces, we can find ways of inserting chemical or genetic blockades to force the virus to put on its brakes. Recently, scientists discovered an AIDS medication called 3TC that does exactly that for hepatitis B—a good sign that our knowledge of virology (the study of viruses) is improving rapidly.

Recently, two laboratories isolated a special part of the hepatitis C virus called protease. Researchers anticipate that they will be able to develop specific drugs that will inhibit this protease and be highly effective in treating hepatitis C. Similar types of drugs are currently used to treat HIV patients and have been effective in clearing HIV from blood and tissue. The future holds much promise.

As a doctor, I'm excited when a patient conquers and clears the hepatitis C virus. Many patients fail to clear the virus but still have other victories along the way. Any illness, especially a chronic one, tests a person's limits. My hope is that the following chapters will help you learn more about hepatitis C and make you more comfortable with your choices and challenges from day to day.

The beginning of wisdom is to call things by their right names.
Chinese proverb

Reference

1. Peter Radetsky, *The Invisible Invaders: Viruses and the Scientists Who Pursue Them* (Boston: Little Brown and Co., 1994) p. 8.

2

When You Have Hepatitis C
Understanding the Diagnosis:
Blood Tests and Biopsies

For two years I knew there was something wrong. I was tired all the time. In a weird way it was almost a relief when my doctor came up with a diagnosis. Finally, I knew I wasn't crazy or a hypochondriac.

But hepatitis C? My skin wasn't yellow, and I didn't feel that bad. I blurted out the first thing that came into my head: "Did you make a mistake?"

Kevin

"BUT I FEEL FINE!" many of my patients say when I tell them that blood tests show they have hepatitis C. They often follow with, "Are you sure?" All of us, when we hear upsetting news, have the same reaction. A layer of protective denial shelters us from absorbing the news too quickly. We feel almost numb. Then, as our bodies adapt to the increased stress, we start to question. Could there be a mistake?

This chapter answers that question and many others about the testing process for hepatitis C from the time you are diagnosed through the years of ongoing care. It covers the following topics:

Can Diagnostic Tests Be Wrong?

Although current tests for hepatitis C are very good, none are perfectly accurate. Every test has a low rate of both false positives and false negatives. To understand why, you have to learn a little bit about the way these tests work. Most of the tests for hepatitis C measure antibodies that your body produces against the virus. Newer tests can actually measure the virus itself (RNA), quantitate levels of the virus, and determine the viral subtype.

When hepatitis C invades the body, your immune system, which is like an army, sends protein "soldiers" into your bloodstream. These proteins are *antibodies*, and they shape themselves to match molecules (called antigens) on the surface of the virus. The antibodies attach themselves to the hepatitis C virus, and your body's white blood cells then move in to destroy the invader.

The two primary blood tests used to detect hepatitis C, ELISA and RIBA assays, work by reacting to hepatitis C antibodies.

ELISA I. A few months after the discovery of hepatitis C in 1989, ELISA I became available. It detected the antibody for an antigen named C-100. However, ELISA I produced many false-positive results and did not detect the virus in about one-third of cases. If you were diagnosed from 1989 to 1992, and you were never treated or retested, you may want to ask your doctor about ELISA II.

ELISA II. In 1993 scientists developed a more sensitive test called ELISA II. This improved assay contains *four* antigens produced by hepatitis C, so it is more sensitive and specific with fewer false-positive reactions.

Let's go back to the original question, "Can my diagnosis be wrong?" There are still some false-positive reports with ELISA II. Nonspecific antibodies may bind to the hepatitis C antigens or react against an enzyme (superoxide dismutase) found in about 3 percent of the normal population. It's a problem of mistaken identity. A positive result with ELISA could be a reaction against the enzyme and not hepatitis C antigens.

RIBA. If you test positive by ELISA II, your doctor may decide to confirm the results with RIBA. RIBA is an assay that determines exactly which hepatitis C antigens the antibodies in your blood are reacting to. If your reaction is only against superoxide dismutase, and not against the hepatitis C antigens, you don't have hepatitis C. If you react against two or more hepatitis C antigens, you do have hepatitis C. If you react against only one antigen, then you may or may not have hepatitis C. RNA tests can sort out this diagnostic dilemma.

Testing Limits. The above diagnostic tests measure your antibody response to the hepatitis C virus. They don't measure the virus itself. Antibodies may stay in your body even after you've cleared the virus. A positive result, therefore, means one of the following:

1. You've got an ongoing infection with hepatitis C.
2. You've been exposed to hepatitis C but you're currently immune. (Some lucky people apparently do fight off HCV on their own, as many as 15 percent; others may respond to interferon and clear the virus.)
3. You're an infant who received the antibody from your hepatitis-C-infected mother through the placenta. The transferred antibodies usually clear within three months, unless the baby also becomes infected.

I found out I had hepatitis C when I donated blood and got a letter from the blood bank. What a shock! I didn't go to a doctor right away because I had recently changed jobs and I was waiting for my new insurance papers to arrive. So I joined a support group to find out what the heck I had.

They were all talking about a new test that measured the amount of virus in your blood. It was used for research experiments and had just become available for the public. After my insurance papers came, I had the test done and it came back negative—zero—nothing. Do I have hepatitis C or not?

Karen

HCV-RNA Assays. Karen tested positive for hepatitis C antibodies. But when she took a test that directly measured the virus in her blood, called the HCV-RNA assay, she tested negative. Does she have hepatitis C or not?

To answer the question, you need to know that there are two kinds of assays: (1) PCR (Polymerase Chain Reaction) and (2) Branched-Chain DNA.

1. **PCR Assay.** This method is often used for monitoring people on interferon therapy to see if they are clearing the virus. It is not yet known which of the newly developed PCR assays are the most sensitive or specific. Some labs claim that their assay is so sensitive that it can detect as few as 100 virus particles per milliliter of blood. Current assays are expensive (of-

ten more than $250) and may be cumbersome to use on a large number of samples.

2. **Branched-Chain DNA Assay.** Chiron Corporation produced the Branched-Chain DNA method. Although the method is easier to apply to a large number of samples, it is relatively insensitive. It measures HCV-RNA levels only above 200,000 viral particles per milliliter.

Getting back to Karen's case, a PCR quantitative assay can give different results at different times. Sensitivity and reproducibility of PCR assays vary among laboratories, and viral levels in your body may fluctuate. Either may have occurred in Karen's case. Perhaps she has only a small amount of virus in her blood, so small the test cannot detect it. If she is retested for HCV-RNA, the virus might show up. On the other hand, Karen may have been exposed to hepatitis C and cleared it. The positive antibody reflects her previous immune response to the virus. (Post-transfusion data suggests that as many as 15 percent of patients with acute hepatitis C will clear their infection.)

Here's Hedy's experience:

> *The first time I had a PCR test, the results were mathematical gobbledygook: 5.5×10^6 viral particles per milliliter of blood. What does that mean? Is that high? Low? It turns out that it's medium—a little above the mean.*
>
> *I wanted to hear that I had a low level of virus. For days, I was quietly depressed. Many months later, I had another PCR. I was prepared to hear I had the same or higher results. To my surprise, the viral count was down, way down. I was glad, but it also made me begin to accept how little control I have over this virus.*

What do the numbers mean? What's high and what's low? Anything less than 1×10^6 is low. A number greater than 3×10^6 is considered high.

Genotyping. After you've gone through these tests, you may want to know your genotype. Widely used for research, genotype testing recently became available to practicing physicians through commercial laboratories.

The hepatitis C virus is really a whole family of viruses with six major subtypes. In the United States, types 1a and 1b account for 70 to 75 percent of cases. Different subtypes predominate elsewhere in the world.

Why is this important? We've learned that the subtypes respond differently to therapy. Subtypes 1a and 1b are relatively resistant to interferon. By contrast, subtypes 2 and 3 seem to respond better. However, we still can't accurately predict success or failure of therapy in an individual based on the HCV subtype. I've seen patients with all subtypes respond to interferon therapy.

Radiologic Imaging. Don't be alarmed if your doctor orders an ultrasound or a CT scan. The tests are non-invasive and give information about your liver.

Ultrasound. Ultrasonography is a safe and painless way to investigate the size, structure, and the vascular (blood) supply of the liver. It's the preferred radiologic technique for an initial assessment for liver tumors.

Ultrasonic waves penetrate the body tissues and a recording device picks up reflected sound waves that yield an image of the liver. You can compare it to exploring for oil by using seismographic recordings of the earth's formations.

Here's what ultrasound helps find out: liver size and texture and the size of bile ducts and blood vessels. Doppler probes added to ultrasound can detect direction and rates of blood flow in vessels going to and from the liver. Your physician may order ultrasound to pinpoint the liver's location just before a biopsy.

CT Scan. Unlike ultrasound, computed tomography (CT scan) uses a highly sophisticated X-ray machine to scan the internal organs with minimal radiation. CT scans are used to confirm the findings of ultrasound and to get a clearer view because, unlike ultrasound, CT scans aren't blocked by air in the bowel. The scans are also more standardized and much less dependent on the expertise of the technician performing the test. CT scans define the size and texture of the liver and can detect an early liver tumor (see Figure 2A).

FIGURE 2A. CT SCANS OF NORMAL LIVER, CIRRHOTIC LIVER, AND LIVER TUMOR (HEPATOMA)

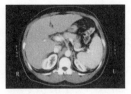 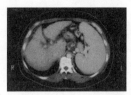 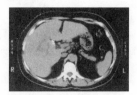

NONCIRRHOTIC   CIRRHOTIC   LIVER CANCER
                                                     (HEPATOMA)

LEGEND 2A: CT scans are specialized radiologic tests that allow one to peer inside the abdomen. The image on the left demonstrates a normal liver and spleen. The middle panel depicts a liver with a knobby irregular surface and an enlarged spleen in a cirrhotic patient. The image to the right shows a liver cancer (hepatoma) in the middle of the liver. The patient with the cancer was treated by chemoembolization of the tumor and liver transplantation and is currently alive without evidence of tumor.

Liver Biopsy. Just the word "biopsy" strikes fear into people's hearts, but it's an essential part of your treatment. Only a biopsy can give your doctor a true idea of the condition of your liver. You need a biopsy for two reasons:

1. It confirms the diagnosis and rules out other disorders, such as granulomatous liver disease, infections, or biliary tract disorders. Liver biopsy along with ultrasound or a CT scan can be used to pinpoint the site of a lesion and rule out liver cancers or lymphoma.
2. It establishes the stage and degree of activity of hepatitis C. Typically, chronic viral hepatitis passes in sequence from a mild inflammatory stage to fibrosis and, later, cirrhosis. Biopsies may be done over many years to record the progression. Once cirrhosis has developed, there is little reason to continue the biopsies.

Years ago, liver biopsies were often performed under general anesthesia and required a short hospital stay. Today it's an outpatient procedure that literally takes *seconds*. In fact, you'll spend most of your time getting ready for the biopsy. However, it is invasive, and you will be asked to sign an informed consent form. It's a good idea to select a doctor who frequently performs this procedure and is very familiar with it. Biopsies may be performed every three to five years.

> *I didn't tell my wife I tested positive for hepatitis C; I didn't want to worry her. When my doctor ordered a biopsy and explained what it was, I figured "piece of cake."*
>
> *I took the afternoon off from work and drove myself to the hospital and back, but we had tickets to a play that evening. I got back home with no time to rest. The play was a bad idea. We had to leave early, and the whole story came tumbling out. That was the end of my macho phase.*
>
> *Kevin*

As you can see from Kevin's story, it's helpful to plan a quiet, restful period after a biopsy. In my experience, most patients' fears come from not knowing what to expect. Here's how the procedure goes:

Your physician examines you carefully to decide exactly where to place the biopsy needle and cleanse the skin with iodine or an antiseptic solution. Then you'll get a local anesthetic, as you do at the dentist's, at the spot where the biopsy needle will be placed. Some doctors also prescribe intravenous benzodiazepine with a narcotic to lessen the anxiety and discomfort.

You'll feel strong pressure when the needle is inserted, but the whole procedure takes only a few seconds for a small core of tissue to be obtained. Then you'll be rolled onto your right side to help control any bleeding from the surface of the liver. You'll stay in the procedure area for two to four hours for observation. If you're stable, with no symptoms, you'll be discharged. Otherwise, you may be admitted to the hospital for observation.

After performing biopsies on hundreds of patients, I've seen very few complications. Reported rates vary from 1 percent to 0.1 percent. If the most common complication occurs, bleeding from the surface of the liver, the patient may require transfusions or even an operation. In rare cases, the biopsy needle may pierce another organ, such as the bowel, gallbladder, kidney, or lung. Death occurs very rarely, in less than one in 1,000 cases.

Interpreting Biopsy Results

Your doctor will tell you the results of your biopsy in terms of histologic stages. Histology means the examination of tissue under the microscope. There are four histologic stages in liver injury due to hepatitis C:

- **Stage I** is characterized by inflammation without the development of any scar tissue.
- **Stage II** features include inflammation with early scarring (fibrosis) in one zone (portal) of the liver.
- **Stage III** shows bridging of the fibrosis between adjacent portal tracts.
- **Stage IV** is cirrhosis (advanced scarring with loss of normal liver architecture).

Histologic stages don't correspond very well to the duration of infection. For example, a patient with slowly progressive disease may maintain an early histologic stage for many years or even decades. Another patient may progress to cirrhosis in less than a decade. The stages of liver damage are distinctive under the microscope (see Figure 2B).

Physicians use certain specific terms when interpreting liver biopsies from patients with hepatitis C. Here's a quick translation:

Stage of Disease	Terminology
Early stage, mild activity (I)	Chronic Persistent Hepatitis C or Mild Chronic Active Hepatitis C
Intermediate stage (II or III)	Chronic Active Hepatitis C with Fibrosis
Advanced stage (IV)	Cirrhosis

FIGURE 2B. HISTOLOGIC STAGES OF HEPATITIS C

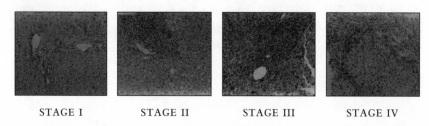

| STAGE I | STAGE II | STAGE III | STAGE IV |

LEGEND 2B: This figure demonstrates the progressive microscopic changes that may occur in livers infected with hepatitis C. Stage I shows only mild inflammation in the portal tract; stage II exhibits more inflammation with spread of fibrosis (scar tissue) into adjacent liver cells; stage III implies that fibrosis has spread between portal tracts; stage IV is cirrhosis with formation of nodules.

After the Diagnosis, Then What? Tests and More Tests

Life with hepatitis C means lots of blood tests to monitor your condition. Have you ever wondered what the numbers really mean? If medico-babble is getting in your way, simplify. Read the next few pages to review the warning signals of five basic blood tests:

1. enzymes
2. bilirubin
3. albumin
4. clotting factors
5. complete blood count

Doctors test blood so frequently in viral hepatitis patients because blood tests warn of changes. The most informative tests "dip" into this bloodstream to measure liver injury (enzymes) or assess liver function (bilirubin, albumin, clotting factors, complete blood count). At first, you may feel intimidated by medical terminology, acronyms, and numbers, but learning about these basic tests will help you understand your doctor's interpretation of results. Hedy says:

Who ever heard of this complicated stuff before hepatitis C? At first, I kept track of my liver enzymes religiously, writing each ALT and AST score on a yellow legal pad. I ignored the other numbers on the lab report.

Now I understand that the other function tests let me know how my liver is coping with the infection—like looking into the liver without a microscope. I always ask for a copy of my test results, and I keep my own file. It helps me feel as if I'm doing all I can on my end.

Liver Enzymes. A liver cell produces proteins, called enzymes, that live within the cell or its membranes. In a way, you can think of your liver as a powerful chemical factory; it changes raw materials into the substances your body needs. Enzymes are catalysts that help a liver cell do its job of creating the specific chemical changes that give your body fuel to live. Here are the names of the enzymes you need to remember:

• ALT (SGPT)—alanine aminotransferase
• AST (SGOT)—aspartate aminotransferase
• GGT—gamma-glutamyl transferase
• alkaline phosphatase

By measuring their level in your blood, doctors can monitor ongoing liver injury. Why? Under normal conditions, the level of these enzymes in your bloodstream is relatively low. But when liver cells are injured, destroyed, or die, the cell becomes leaky, and the enzymes escape into the blood that's circulating through the liver. When the cell is injured, liver enzyme levels in the blood rise. Massive liver injury is associated with marked increases in ALT; mild injury may be associated with mild— or even no—increase in ALT. The correlation is strongest at earlier stages of hepatitis C, before the development of cirrhosis. However, once cirrhosis occurs, ALT levels may not be high; therefore, ALT is no longer a good indicator of further liver damage.

What do the numbers mean? Table 1 shows normal and ab-

TABLE 1. NORMAL AND ABNORMAL VALUES
FOR LABORATORY TESTS

Test	Normal Range	Abnormal Range	
		Mild to Moderate	Severe
Liver Enzymes			
AST	< 40 IU/L	40–200	> 200
ALT	< 40 IU/L	40–200	> 200
GGT	< 60 IU/L	60–200	> 200
Alkaline Phosphatase	<112 IU/L	112–300	> 300
Liver Function Tests			
Bilirubin	< 1.2 mg/dl	1.2–2.5	> 2.5
Albumin	3.5–4.5 g/dl	3.0–3.5	< 3.0
Prothrombin Time	< 14 seconds	14–17	> 17
Blood Count			
WBC	> 6000	3000–6000	< 3000
HCT	> 40	35–40	< 35
Platelets	> 150,000	100,000–150,000	< 100,000

KEY:
IU = International Units
l = liter
dl = deciliter
mg = milligrams
AST (SGOT) = aspartate aminotransferase
ALT (SGPT) = alanine aminotransferase
GGT = gamma-glutamyl transferase
WBC = white blood count
HCT = hematocrit (percentage of blood occupied
      by red blood cells)

normal test values. Blood test patterns relate somewhat to the type of liver injury. Typical hepatitis C patients show increases in ALT and AST but little or no increase in GGT and alkaline phosphatase. Those with cirrhosis or who have an underlying disorder of the biliary tract (the ducts that drain bile from the liver into the intestine) may have modest elevations in GGT and alkaline phosphatase. In some unusual cases of hepatitis C I have even seen a predominant elevation in GGT.

Patients tend to focus on their ALT and AST counts, but other tests are more important in measuring the health of your liver.

Bilirubin

After the birth of my second child—a caesarean delivery that required blood transfusions—I learned I was infected with hepatitis C. My AST and ALT counts were only slightly elevated. The most important thing to me was raising my little boys as best I could for as long as I could. I wanted them to know their mother. So I decided to delay treatment and watch my bloodwork every three months.

I made it to my youngest son's ninth birthday when the test pattern changed. "Your bilirubin is up," my doctor said. "It's time to start interferon."

There went the PTA and baking cupcakes—but I did respond to interferon. A good trade.

Jill

When red blood cells complete their life cycle and break down naturally in your body, they produce a yellow pigment that's passed to the liver and excreted into bile. Bile helps your body digest food, but the pigment, which has no digestive function, is called bilirubin. Blood levels of bilirubin tend to fluctuate in patients with hepatitis, although a prolonged persistent elevation in bilirubin usually means severe liver dysfunction and possibly cirrhosis.

Here's why. Most of the time, the body produces as many red blood cells as it breaks down, so you produce a constant amount of bilirubin. However, if your blood cells break down more rapidly (hemolysis) or your liver function becomes impaired, the bilirubin levels in your blood rise.

Your liver has to go to work to take up the excess bilirubin into the liver cell, metabolize it to make it more water-soluble for excretion into bile, and send it through special passages and ducts into the intestine. Microbes in the gut continue to metabolize the bilirubin until you expel it. (Stercobilin, a brown pigment derived from bilirubin, creates the dark brown color of feces.)

When the liver fails to eliminate bilirubin from the blood, the skin and whites of the eyes turn yellow (jaundice), urine darkens, and the color of the bowel movement lightens. In case you've wondered, now you know why your doctor asks you probing questions about the color of your feces.

Albumin. Albumin is another protein synthesized (manufactured) by the liver. Liver cells secrete albumin to maintain the volume of blood in arteries and veins. When albumin levels drop to extremely low levels, fluid may leak out of the blood vessels into the surrounding tissues. This causes swelling, known as edema. Normal albumin levels range between 3.5 to 4.5 grams/deciliter. Usually, edema occurs when levels drop below 2.5 grams/deciliter.

Unlike liver enzyme increases, which occur within hours to days of the liver injury, albumin levels don't fall unless there has been chronic progressive liver injury for at least one month or more. This is because albumin has a long residence time in the plasma; its half life is approximately 30 days. A decrease in serum albumin, therefore, reflects a slowly progressive, ongoing reduction in the liver's ability to synthesize this protein.

Be aware that there are non-liver reasons for albumin to decrease and your physician will take these into account when interpreting test results. Nonetheless, a significant sustained decrease in serum albumin may mean poor liver function and cirrhosis of the liver. Patients with very low albumin counts may need to be considered for liver transplantation.

Clotting Factors. Remember our comparison of the liver to a chemical factory? The liver also synthesizes many proteins that maintain normal blood clotting. Prothrombin time (PT) is the name of the most common test that measures a combination of blood clotting factors. If your prothrombin time increases, it means your liver isn't creating enough factors, so it takes your blood longer to clot.

Unlike albumin, clotting factors can decrease rapidly—within days, or even hours, of a severe liver injury. In severe cases, clotting disturbances may signal the need for an early transplant. In patients with chronic hepatitis and chronic liver disease, a prolonged prothrombin time can be a warning that the liver is having trouble with its synthetic functions.

Typically, doctors will administer vitamin K, a vitamin essential for normal clotting factors, to determine whether the clotting disorder is reversible. Patients who have persistent, prolonged elevations in prothrombin time that don't respond to vitamin K may need to be considered for liver transplantation.

Complete Blood Count. The complete blood count test can be a detection system for liver scarring. Here's how. Blood from your spleen flows through your liver via the portal vein. When the liver becomes scarred, it creates resistance to this blood flow (called portal hypertension), and the blood may back up into the spleen. When this happens, the spleen enlarges and traps blood elements, removing them from circulation and lowering blood counts.

Although all components of the blood count may decrease, those most sensitive to this condition are the white blood cell and platelet counts. Patients with portal hypertension from cirrhosis of the liver often have low counts. Similarly, patients may have an enlarged spleen, resulting from severe cirrhotic disease, and may need to be considered for liver transplantation.

Testing, Testing. In the past few years, I've seen the development of wonderful new tests that help monitor your health. But all too often I find that patients feel shut out by the complicated language of test results. Don't worry if you didn't absorb every detail. Use these pages as a reference guide.

Ask for copies of your tests. When you have questions, look them up in these pages. Often, your physician can calm your fears if you voice them. Talk with your doctor.

Knowledge is power.

Francis Bacon

3

Why Me?
What About Them?

How You Got Infected and
How to Avoid Infecting Others

*When my doctor told me I had hepatitis C, I said, "No way!
You've got the wrong blood test. It's got to be some kind of mix-
up."*

*I've never had a transfusion or done drugs. Even when I had
my ears pierced, it was with those disposable studs. I mean, I'm a
really cautious person. What did I do to deserve this?*

Juliana

WHEN YOU'RE DEALING with a serious illness,
it's the most human thing in the world to ask, "Why
me? What did I do to get hepatitis C?"

The answer is both simple and complex. Most likely you acquired hepatitis C when you came into contact with blood infected with the virus, and it gained entry into your bloodstream.

The complicating factor is that as many as 40 percent of people with hepatitis C fail to report the way in which they were ex-

posed to infectious blood. And, unlike hepatitis A or B, patients rarely recall a severe initial attack of the disease to mark the time of infection.

How did *you* get hepatitis C? And how can you avoid giving the virus to others? We'll discuss ways to protect your family and friends. In addition, we'll provide up-to-date summaries of documented ways that hepatitis C is transmitted, including:

- Intravenous Drug Abuse
- Transfusion of Blood or Blood-Products
    Coronary Bypass Surgery
    Hemophilia
- Needle-Stick Accidents
- Tattooing and Body Piercing
- Sharing Sharp Instruments
- Birth and Delivery (rare)
- Sexual Transmission (rare)
- Organ Transplantation (rare)
- How Can I Avoid Infecting Others?

Intravenous Drug Abuse

What's the most direct way to get hepatitis C? Inoculate the virus from infected blood into your own bloodstream. That's why one of the most common risk factors is a history of using intravenous illicit drugs. Many drug addicts share needles. They spread hepatitis among themselves and maintain a pool of infected people. Studies suggest that more than 75 percent of current or past users of intravenous drugs may have hepatitis C.

Although heavy drug abusers may be at greatest risk, many people who have hepatitis C report only rare experimentation in the distant past. Unfortunately, the wise decision to stop taking drugs doesn't erase the risk from prior use.

I'm a therapist. People come to me for help with drug abuse. But 20 years ago, when I was a college freshman, I went a little

wild. For the first time I was away from home, and I did some
drugs. And yes, I shared needles once or twice. If only I could go
back and change what I did. . . .

Jake

When I question patients about how they got the virus, they usually don't have a clue. I ask them if they've had transfusions or experimented with intravenous drugs. They're shocked. "Can that do it?" they'll say. "It was only once or twice."

When we don't know how the person got hepatitis C, we call it "sporadic" or "community acquired." Some doctors think that most of these cases are due to prior use of intravenous drugs. Patients who are otherwise healthy, employed, and raising their families are stunned to hear they have hepatitis C. They can't believe the diagnosis relates to a past, seemingly insignificant experiment so long ago.

"I don't know how I could get hepatitis C from sharing needles. I was always so careful about cleaning them," patients often say. But to understand how contamination occurs, you have to appreciate how concentrated the virus is in the blood of infected patients.

The average patient with chronic hepatitis C has a blood concentration of the virus of two million particles per milliliter of whole blood. That's equivalent to 2,000 particles of virus in the amount of blood that would sit on the head of a small stickpin. With this concentration it's easy to see that wiping or rinsing a needle with water or salt solutions won't remove all the virus particles. Indeed, a large amount of virus may remain on the needle.

A concentrated solution of hydrogen peroxide will kill or inactivate the virus, and cleaning needles with this solution may reduce the risk of transmission. It won't protect you, however, if cleaning is superficial, such as a quick rinse, or if the internal chamber of the needle is not irrigated and the syringe and all its external and internal parts are not cleansed. Some people rely on others to clean a syringe and don't realize that it's not done thoroughly.

We Americans face a tremendous public health problem from illegal IV drug use. According to Drug Strategies, a nonprofit re-

search institute, since 1980, U.S. federal, state, and local govern-
ments have spent about $20 billion a year on anti-drug programs
(twice as much as the federal government spends annually for biomedical research). Yet there are still an estimated 12 million
Americans who admit they use illicit drugs at least once a month.
When interviewed by the 1995 National Household Survey on
Drug Abuse, an estimated 2,723,000 Americans over the age of 12
said they had injected drugs at some time during their lives.

On a personal level, the risk factor rises each time you use
drugs. If you shoot up once, you may or may not get hepatitis C.
But if you shoot up many times, you can almost count on it. The
best way to avoid the risk is to avoid illicit intravenous drugs and
to teach the next generation to avoid this dangerous behavior.

Transfusion of Blood or Blood Products

The risk of getting hepatitis C from the transfusion of blood or
blood products has been steadily declining since the mid-1980s.
Before 1986, there was virtually no screening of blood donors for
hepatitis C (then called Non A/Non B), except for sporadic ALT
testing. In 1986, blood banks throughout the United States began
screening blood donors for hepatitis by measuring ALT (a liver
enzyme) and hepatitis B core antibody. Use of these tests by blood
banks reduced the risk of acquiring hepatitis C by transfusion one
hundred-fold.

Two recent, widely quoted studies (see Table 3) reported the

TABLE 3. RISK OF POST-TRANSFUSION HEPATITIS C

Era	Test screening	Cases per 10,000 units transfused
Prior to 1986	None	45
1986–1990	ALT, HBcAb (HIV-Ab, 1985)	19
1990–1991	HCV-Ab, EIA 1	3
1992–1993	HCV-Ab, EIA 2	0.4

per unit transfusion risk for the screening procedures. As you can see, scientists developed a test for hepatitis C in 1990 and then improved it in 1992. As a result, the risk of contracting the virus from transfusions went way down.

> *I'd never been sick a day in my life. Then in 1974, I had a car crash and received multiple blood transfusions.*
>
> *After the accident, things were never the same. I used to play ball, but heck—it got to where I was always so tired, I could barely go to the games. Forget playing in them.*
>
> *Terry*

You may be wondering if there is currently any risk at all. If a blood donor was recently exposed to hepatitis C, he may be in the "window period" before antibodies form and will therefore test negative. The virus, however, is circulating in his blood and will be passed on to a recipient if the blood is used for transfusion. For this reason, statisticians estimate the risk of infection as extremely low, but there's no such thing as zero risk.

Certain medical procedures and operations were particularly associated with risk of acquiring hepatitis C due to the large number of transfusions required. These included hemodialysis, coronary artery bypass or heart surgery, lung resection, and major abdominal surgery.

Hemophilia. People with hemophilia lack certain clotting factors in their blood. In the past hemophiliacs were treated with plasma from a large number of donors. The plasma was combined and treated to extract those clotting factors.

Until the mid-1980s, hemophiliacs were at extreme risk for getting hepatitis B and HIV. Therefore, scientists pasteurized the clotting factor for hemophiliacs and this treatment inactivated the hepatitis C virus. When tests for hepatitis C became available in 1990, studies showed that hemophiliacs treated with unpasteurized preparations had an 80 to 90 percent chance of having hepatitis C, while those who received the pasteurized preparation had an extremely low risk, approaching zero percent. Today, current therapy often uses synthesized or genetically engineered clotting products with a zero risk of transmitting hepatitis C.

Needle-Stick Accidents

Health care workers face an occupational hazard: needle-stick accidents. Because many hospitalized patients and people who frequent emergency rooms have hepatitis, medical personnel run high risks if they accidentally get stuck with an infected needle, which can easily pierce rubber gloves.

Here's Hedy:

> I watched the lab tech tie a rubber band around my arm. "I have hepatitis C," I said, noticing that she wore only one glove, so she could probe my skin to check for a 'good' vein. "You might want to put on another glove."
>
> "That's okay," she said, smiling. "I've got hepatitis C, too."

In one study of an inner city emergency room at Johns Hopkins Hospital in Baltimore, MD., 24 percent of 2,523 patients over age 15 were infected with at least one of three viruses: HIV (6 percent), hepatitis B (5 percent), or hepatitis C (18 percent). Eighty-three percent of the intravenous drug users, 21 percent of the people who had transfusions, and 21 percent of the homosexual male patients had hepatitis C. Of all the patients who were bleeding and who had invasive procedures performed, 30 percent had at least one virus.

This study shows the potential exposure of medical personnel to hepatitis C infection. HIV testing alone failed to identify 87 percent of those who had hepatitis B and 80 percent of patients with hepatitis C.

> When I started my career as a medical technician, I got a needle stick. They gave me gamma globulin, but the supply was tainted until 1990. Then two years ago, they detected hepatitis C. I was really sick with infected fluid in my legs, and I was hemorrhaging. They gave me 25 units of blood.

Out of five people in our lab, three ended up with hepatitis C, but mine is the only one that became active. My doctor calls it "a thief in the night."

Erica

Fortunately, the risk of acquiring hepatitis C after a needle stick is relatively low. In two studies with a total of 201 cases of needle-stick accidents involving hepatitis C patients, transmission occurred in only 5 percent.

The best measure of virus in the blood is HCV-RNA (see Chapter 2, PCR assays). None of the RNA-negative patients transmitted HCV to the staff, but seven cases (10 percent) of hepatitis C developed in medical personnel who got the needle stick from an RNA-positive patient. These limited results suggest that health care workers receiving needle sticks from RNA-positive patients are at greatest risk.

How do we treat a person who has a needle-stick accident? No one has conducted a well-studied approach to treatment. Although immune serum globulin is commonly administered, we haven't proven its ability to prevent hepatitis C. In contrast, interferon may be useful in preventing the hepatitis from becoming chronic.

I currently recommend that all individuals sustaining a needle stick from an HCV antibody-positive patient be monitored in the following ways: ALT monthly for six months; HCV-Ab (EIA2) at baseline, six months, and 12 months. People who develop elevated ALT or positive HCV antibody should undergo RNA testing and be considered for interferon therapy.

Tattooing and Body Piercing

Tattooing and body piercing are ancient rites in many cultures. In this country, we're witnessing a recent surge of interest in "body art." The practice of tattooing is particularly common in the military and among gang members and prisoners. It's also becoming an accepted cosmetic practice.

Celebrities have popularized the trend. Comedian Roseanne

and ex-husband Tom Arnold had each other's names tattooed on their backsides. Famous athletes have decorated their bodies, including Mike Peluso's tattoo of the Stanley Cup and Steve Everitt's bleeding dagger. Unfortunately, even the most benign-appearing tattooing may have its dark side (see Figure 3). Viral hepatitis, mainly hepatitis B, is the best documented infection transmitted by tattoos in the 20th century. Two epidemiologic studies implicate tattooing in the transmission of hepatitis C.

Here's a switch. I'm a tattoo artist, and last year I found out I have hepatitis C. I have antibodies to hepatitis B, too. My joints hurt so much, I can't work. I feel like I'm sliding down the evolutionary scale, because I can't move my opposable thumbs.

I'm sure I got hepatitis from a needle stick. Fifteen years ago, who wore gloves?

Peter

FIGURE 3. HEPATITIS C PATIENT WITH TATTOO

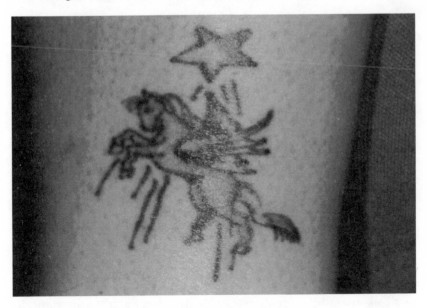

LEGEND: This seemingly innocuous tattoo may have been a source of transmission of hepatitis C to this patient.

Nine percent of males and 1 percent of females in the United States get tattoos—with peak ages between 14 and 22. And tattoos are common in certain groups at high risk for hepatitis C and other viral infections: intravenous drug abusers, gang members, prostitutes, and prisoners. In one study 65 percent of prisoners had tattoos.

> *This flag on my arm—I was young and in the Navy. What did I know? Now I'm told that there are certified tattoo artists, and if you go to someone reputable, everything is sterilized.*
> *Well, too late for me. It wasn't like that in Hong Kong.*
>
> *Jerry*

Tattooing involves shaving the skin, placing ink on it, then pushing the ink through the skin with a needle gun. A small amount of bleeding is common. The problem is that sterilization techniques vary, and home-tattooing kits may contain inadequate methods for sterilization.

Body piercing of the earlobes, nose, lips, and other areas also breaks the skin. Therefore, the principles and risk of transmission of hepatitis C are the same as in tattooing.

Sharing Sharp Instruments

Family and friends who live with hepatitis C patients don't appear to have an increased risk of getting the virus. Nonetheless, you should take care to prevent your blood, which contains hepatitis C, from inoculating another person accidentally.

> *Yesterday I found my oldest son, a teenager, standing in front of the bathroom mirror and trying to shave for the first time. I got so scared. My husband has hepatitis C.*
> *Why didn't we see how fast our son was growing? Why didn't we warn him not to borrow his dad's razor?*
>
> *Jan*

Talk to family members and explain why it's important to avoid sharing razor blades, nailclippers, scissors, and toothbrushes. These measures are just good hygiene; it's also sensible to bandage any cuts or abrasions and to safely dispose of menstrual pads and tampons.

In my clinical experience I have seen only one case where transmission of viral hepatitis (hepatitis B, in this instance) from brother to sister occurred because they commonly shared a shaving razor blade.

Birth and Delivery

If you have hepatitis C and you're pregnant or planning a family, of course you're concerned about giving birth to a healthy baby. The period of risk occurs at delivery when the mother's and baby's blood may become intermixed. Mothers with hepatitis C who are otherwise healthy rarely transmit the virus to their newborns. The chance of transmitting hepatitis C from mother to baby is less than 5 percent. In contrast, mothers with HIV who are also infected with hepatitis C may transmit hepatitis C to their babies as often as 50 percent of the time.

Mothers with hepatitis C often ask whether they can transmit the virus to their baby through breast feeding. Current studies do not allow us to draw a definite conclusion. However, existing information suggests that hepatitis C is rarely—if ever—transmitted to an infant through breast milk. Even though hepatitis C may be detected in breast milk, it's likely that the baby's digestive juices and enzymes would destroy the virus.

Sexual Transmission

This is one of the most sensitive and troubling topics for patients. The risk of getting hepatitis C through sexual contact is minimal, but some spouses are wary. Trust dissolves, the gap widens, and the couple can end up in divorce court.

It's just as hard for singles. How do you start an intimate relationship without being honest about hepatitis C? And how will the other person react?

I'm single, and I'm not the smoothest, slickest character around. It's always been hard for me to meet women. Now I have to tell them I have hepatitis C. When should I tell them? Will they want to have anything to do with me?

Russ

I'm feeling low, depressed. I was dating this guy, and the relationship was going well. It felt right. Then he broke up with me two days ago. I'm trying not to be paranoid—I mean it could have happened anyway—but he broke up with me a week after I told him I had hepatitis C.

Nancy

Perhaps some solid information will help you come to grips with this issue. Compared to hepatitis B and HIV, hepatitis C circulates in your blood at relatively low levels. It is either not detected or found in low concentrations in body fluids, such as saliva, urine, feces, semen, or vaginal secretions.

The vast majority of sexual partners of patients with hepatitis C test negative for hepatitis C. When a sexual partner does test positive, in most cases this partner has had other risk factors for acquiring hepatitis C, such as intravenous drug use or exposure to blood or blood products. Here's the important news. In selected couples without other risk factors, it is estimated that no transmission of the virus occurred despite a projected 160,000 sexual exposures.

Another study failed to document any case of sexual transmission of hepatitis C in 50 partners—even after a calculated 713 person-years of exposure through sexual contact. In short, the overall evidence from a wide variety of studies shows that heterosexual transmission of hepatitis C in a stable, single-partner relationship occurs only very rarely.

Sally's diagnosis shocked us. We were completely naive. She worried about giving me hepatitis C until we learned more and got a pretty good handle on it.

We've been cautious, but it's not like I'm terrified to go near her. We've been together six years, and I saw no reason to treat her differently or to change our behavior, because I was already exposed.

Sally felt dirty. I did everything I could to diffuse that. It didn't affect the way I felt about her. I kissed her the day before the diagnosis, so why not kiss her the day after?

Ken

My husband got completely paranoid. When I first found out I had hepatitis C, I wanted him to say, "We'll get through this together," but he didn't. He was really nice for a week, then he started getting hostile. He couldn't handle it. I think a big part of it was that we were getting conflicting information about whether or not you can transmit the virus sexually.

We were having troubles before—and I guess the added strain was too much. During my fifth month of interferon, he left me and our three-year-old daughter.

Danielle

Although sexual transmission in stable heterosexual partnerships rarely occurs, some studies suggest that sexual transmission of hepatitis C may be more frequent in homosexual males or highly promiscuous heterosexuals. Some sexual practices are more traumatic to body tissues. For example, anal intercourse may disrupt the lining of the rectum and allow blood containing hepatitis C to enter the blood of a sexual partner.

Organ Transplantation

Can a person get hepatitis C from a transplanted organ? Yes! If the donor has hepatitis C, the virus will infect the recipient of the donor organ. Two studies address this issue.

In one study, 28 percent of patients who received organs from donors with hepatitis C developed clinical evidence of liver disease during a follow-up period ranging from three months to six-and-a-half years. In a second study, all the recipients who did not have hepatitis C before the transplant, and who received an organ from a hepatitis C donor, developed hepatitis C after the transplant.

In the University of Colorado liver transplant program, we restrict the use of organs from hepatitis C patients to two situations: recipients already infected with hepatitis C or recipients in desperate medical condition who are awaiting a donor organ at the highest urgency status (hospitalized on life support and not likely to survive seven days without a transplant).

Can you, as a hepatitis C patient, donate an organ for transplanting? Yes. Even though you have hepatitis C, you may still be able to donate your organs for transplant. The organs most commonly used are the kidney and liver, but only if the liver shows no active disease or scarring.

How Can I Avoid Infecting Others?

My patients often inquire about protecting friends and family from the virus. Here are some common questions people ask:

Is it okay to kiss and hug my kids? Yes, you can kiss and hug your children, and they can kiss and hug you back. There is no data to suggest that you could infect your children by these actions.

Should I have members of my family tested for hepatitis C? The risk of transmission from you to other family members, including your spouse, is very low and, in general, testing is not necessary. If your spouse or child has elevated liver enzyme tests, then they should be tested for hepatitis C.

Can I cook for my family? What if I cut myself while I'm preparing food? Certainly you can cook for your family. Even if you cut yourself and get blood in the food, it's unlikely that anyone eating the food will get hepatitis C. The enzymes in the digestive tract will destroy or inactivate the virus.

What if my child or friend eats food off my plate or uses my fork? You don't transmit hepatitis C by sharing drinks or food. Hepatitis C is transmitted by contaminated blood entering your bloodstream—not your stomach.

My teenager borrowed my manicure scissors. Is that a problem? I recommend that you avoid sharing sharp instruments.

There is a possibility that if your teenager cut herself on your scissors, she could inoculate herself with blood you might have left on the scissors. Despite this theoretical risk, I don't know any cases where this type of transmission has been documented. However, it's best to avoid sharing all sharp instruments, such as nailclippers, razor blades, toothbrushes, etc.

We've been married for 15 years. Is it safe to have sex? The existing information indicates that sexual transmission between individuals in a stable, single partner, monogamous relationship rarely—if ever—occurs. In addition, people involved in a stable relationship do not need to alter their sexual practices.

I'm single. What should I tell my dates? If you're heterosexual and involved with one partner, my sense is the sexual transmission is so low that it may not be an issue. On the other hand, you have a trust issue that you have to resolve; that may require disclosing your hepatitis C infection. Place the disclosure in the context of knowing that your hepatitis C infection need not fracture or destroy an otherwise promising relationship. Infected males may provide additional protection for their female sexual partners by using latex condoms.

What about French kissing? Oral sex? The details of these types of sexual activity have not been scientifically investigated. If blood barriers (lining of the mouth, lining of the genitalia) are breached, then blood-to-blood transmission may occur.

Should I always use condoms? Latex condoms and safe sex practices are especially suggested for individuals who have multiple sex partners.

Can I have a baby? Nurse my baby? Yes. Mothers who ask these questions are worried about transmitting hepatitis C to their infants. First, the risk of transmission appears to be limited to the time of delivery, when the blood of the mother and infant may become intermixed. Despite this potential route of transmission, less than 4 percent of babies born of mothers with hepatitis C develop the infection.

As stated above, swallowing mother's milk is not likely to be harmful to the infant.

Is it necessary to tell people like my dentist that I have hepatitis C? In my opinion, patients should inform dentists and other health care professionals who need to perform invasive procedures or operations.

Can I be an organ donor? Yes. Some organs from hepatitis C patients are used, particularly for recipients who are critically ill or who already have hepatitis C.

> *We learn geology the morning after the earthquake.*
>
> *Emerson*

4

Learning About Your Liver: Your Body's Chemical Factory

Liver Facts and Liver Disease Symptoms

from Oda al Higado (Ode to the Liver)[1]
by Pablo Neruda
> *. . . navigating*
> *the hidden mysteries,*
> *the alchemist's chamber*
> *of life's microscopic,*
> *echoic, inner oceans . . .*

Translated by Herberto Morales and Will Hochman

IMAGINE A MACHINE that converts food into energy; stores nutrients, fats, and vitamins; makes proteins for blood plasma; and detoxifies poisons. Your liver does all this and more—much more.

But no machine, no matter how powerful, is as versatile as your liver. Even if 75 percent of the liver's mass is taken away, it still functions. And it's the only internal organ that regenerates itself.

This chapter will discuss what the liver looks like, how it functions, and what happens to the liver when it's infected with hepatitis C—including ten warning signals your body sends you when liver function is compromised:

- Liver Facts from Mesopotamian to Modern Times
- A Look at Your Liver
    Appearance
    Under the Microscope
- How Your Liver Works
    Blood
    Bile
    Lymph
    Immune System
    Chemical Factory
    Bilirubin
    ALT, AST, GGT, Alkaline Phosphatase
    Albumin
    Clotting Factors
    Hormones
- Phases of Hepatitis C
    Phase I: Infection
    Phase II: Inflammation
    Phase III: Fibrosis
    Phase IV: Cirrhosis
- Ten Danger Signs of Liver Disease
    Early Warning Signs: #1–#2
        Early Symptoms
        Changes in Liver Functions
    Later Warning Signs of Cirrhosis: #3–#10
        Yellowing of the Skin and Whites of the
            Eyes: Jaundice
        Fluid Buildup: Ascites
        Bleeding: Variceal Hemorrhage
        Mental Confusion: Encephalopathy

Weight Loss
Thinning of Bones (Osteoporosis) and Fractures:
   Metabolic Bone Disease
Blood Clotting Problems: Coagulopathy
Itching: Pruritus
- Other Related Clinical Conditions of Hepatitis C
Kidney Damage
Cryoglobulinemia
Thyroid Disease
Skin Conditions
Autoimmune Conditions

Liver Facts from Mesopotamian to Modern Times

- Mesopotamians didn't know anatomy, but they could see that the liver seemed to be the collecting point for blood, the source of life. Archeologists have found 5,000-year-old Mesopotamian clay models of livers with markings that may have helped priests perform religious rites.
- In ancient cultures animals were sacrificed before battle and their entrails were examined; a healthy blood-red liver was a good omen. Pale livers foretold defeat—an expression that has entered the English language with the term "lily-livered," meaning cowardly.
- In Greek mythology, Prometheus stole fire from the gods and gave it to mankind. Zeus punished him by chaining him to a rock in the mountains. Each day an eagle gnawed at his body, feasting on his liver. Because the liver has such great regenerating capacity, it grew back each night, subjecting Prometheus to an endless ordeal.
- In 1987, a granite sculpture of the liver was unveiled in Ferrol, Spain. The city's coroner, who doubled as the mayor, said that over the years he saw "hundreds of these organs tortured by cocktails, wine, tranquilizers, and other medications . . . but every day, the poor little liver is at work neutralizing and

purifying everything we take in."² As the monument was dedicated, a local poet recited "Oda Al Higado" (Ode to the Liver) by the late Nobel prize-winner, Pablo Neruda.

A Look at Your Liver

Appearance. As a hepatologist, a doctor who studies livers, I sometimes forget that my patients usually don't have a clear idea of what this organ looks like. Here's Hedy:

> As a kid, I hated the sight of blood, never looked at body charts in encyclopedias, and avoided first aid classes. In short, I didn't know where my liver was. Right side or left? High in my chest or low in my gut?
>
> I worried about every ache and pain, sure my condition was getting worse by the minute. So I went to the library and took out some children's books with terrific diagrams and simple explanations.
>
> Finally, I believed my doctor. What I was feeling was heartburn, pure and simple. Learning more about my liver helped me reduce stress and, incidentally, the heartburn.

Learning more about your liver can give you a greater feeling of control and reduce stress, so let's examine this organ—the largest one in your body. The liver weighs about three pounds in an adult male and sits in the upper right of the abdomen, protected by the rib cage (see Figure 4A).

If you've ever gone to the supermarket or butcher, you've seen animal livers. They give you a pretty good idea of what the human liver looks and feels like. Reddish-brown in color, it's shaped like a flattened football with two lobes. The larger lobe lies closest to your right side.

The liver is surrounded by vital organs: diaphragm and lungs above, kidney behind, intestine and colon below.

Major blood vessels serve as conduits to deliver blood to and from the liver. Your blood system transports food, oxygen, and waste. Because your liver is a central depot for so many body func-

FIGURE 4A. ANATOMIC LOCATION OF THE LIVER
IN HUMANS

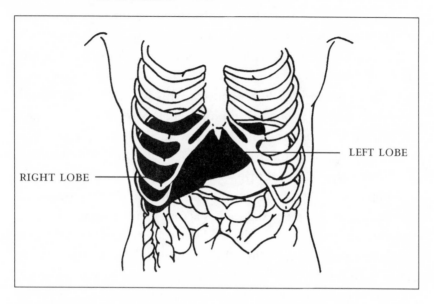

RIGHT LOBE

LEFT LOBE

LEGEND 4A: The liver is located in the right upper quadrant of the abdomen and is protected from external trauma by the rib cage.

tions, it has the largest and most complex blood supply of any organ in the body. In fact, about 1.5 quarts of blood flow through the liver every *minute*.

Like other parts of your body, the liver has an artery to supply it with oxygenated blood (the hepatic artery via the abdominal aorta) and hepatic veins to take blood back to the heart. The hepatic veins join the inferior vena cava, the major vein just below the diaphragm.

In addition to the hepatic artery, the liver has a second source of blood, the portal vein. This vein is responsible for at least two-thirds of liver blood flow and delivers nutrients and toxins absorbed by the intestine to the liver for processing.

Have you ever wondered why livers are a dull red color? It's because the portal vein transports nutrients to the liver in dark, deoxygenated blood.

Speaking of colors, your liver produces up to a quart a day of yellow-green bile, a liquid that looks like motor oil and breaks down fat in foods. Bile flows from the liver into the bile duct, which resembles the branches of a tree. The smallest branches are embedded in the liver while the common bile duct is the tree "trunk."

The common bile duct connects with the gallbladder (which stores bile and is attached to the underside of your liver) through the cystic duct. Then the bile duct continues through the pancreas, where it's joined by the pancreatic duct, and on to the intestine.

Under the Microscope. Tiny units, called lobules, are the building blocks of your liver tissue. Each lobule is a spheroid structure and measures about 0.2 inches across. Under the microscope, you see flat sheets of cube-shaped liver cells (hepatocytes) fanning out from a tiny central vein. Blood flows in the spaces (sinusoids) between the sheets.

Small branches of the hepatic artery (bringing oxygen from the heart) and the portal vein enter the lobule from the side and first deliver blood to the periphery of the lobule (portal area). Blood travels through the lobule toward its center, bathing the hepatocytes with nutrients, chemicals and toxins carried from the intestine. Liver cells have special ways of extracting compounds from blood and metabolizing them—a topic I'll talk about in the next section.

The center of the lobule contains a very fine terminal branch of the hepatic vein. This vein then connects with other branches and "processed" blood flows through the hepatic veins to the inferior vena cava, returning to the heart.

In addition, each liver cell makes and secretes bile to its own tiny attached branch of the biliary system. The liver contains a whole network of these fine tubes that pipe bile to the bile duct and gallbladder.

How Your Liver Works

Knowing how the liver works will help you understand why things go wrong when a virus attacks it. Your liver affects your blood, bile, lymph, immune system, and chemical functions.

Blood. The liver greatly influences the makeup of blood in your body. Blood is composed of plasma (a liquid), red cells, white cells, and platelets. When the liver is diseased, all of these blood components may be affected.

Do you know how your body tissues get oxygen? Red blood cells deliver it. Do you know why wounds clot? Platelets plug bleeding capillaries and vessels. When you have an infection, white blood cells rush to the site as your first line of defense.

The liver receives blood from two sources: two-thirds from the portal vein (which comes from the intestine loaded with nutrients for the liver to process) and one-third from the hepatic artery. The hepatic artery, like all arteries, carries blood loaded with oxygen. About 15 percent of the blood pumped by the heart each minute runs through the liver.

As the liver becomes progressively injured, scar tissue builds up, making it difficult for blood from the portal vein and hepatic artery to flow through the liver. The blood tends to back up into other abdominal vessels and the spleen. As blood backs up in the spleen, cells become trapped and are destroyed—resulting in a decrease in platelets, red cells, and white cells.

Bile. Did you know that cholesterol is an ingredient in bile? Your liver makes bile from water, electrolytes (sodium, potassium, chloride, and others), proteins, organic salts (bilirubin), and lipids (cholesterol, among others). The liver turns compounds that don't dissolve in water into water-soluble substances that are secreted into bile. Toxins (poisons) absorbed from the intestine also circulate in blood to the liver, which extracts, inactivates, and secretes them into bile.

Back to cholesterol. A normal part of our diets, it's made by several cells in our bodies. When too much cholesterol accumulates, cells may alter their functions and even die. If too much cholesterol builds up in blood vessels, you may get hardening of the arteries (atherosclerosis). If it builds up in bile, you may develop gallstones.

Prevention of these complications depends on eliminating excess cholesterol. Your liver is the only organ that breaks down cholesterol into bile acid, secretes it in bile, and removes it from your body for good.

What else does bile do? Simply put, bile helps you absorb fat and vitamins that are dissolved in fat (A, D, E, and K). When disease interrupts this cycle, your body has trouble digesting and absorbing fats and fat-soluble vitamins and getting rid of pigments and toxins.

Lymph. Your liver produces about a quart of lymph a day. Filtered from plasma, it's a protein-rich fluid composed mostly of water and electrolytes. Lymph travels through channels next to the portal vein and joins other major lymph channels in the abdomen. Eventually, the lymph is dumped into the bloodstream.

Any kind of disruption, whether it's disease or congestion of the lymph channels, may mean that large amounts of lymph spill into the abdomen. Although this rarely happens, it may be one reason for swelling of the abdomen due to fluid (ascites).

Immune System. Here's a mouthful: lymphocytes, plasma cells, macrophages, fibroblasts, dendritic cells, and polymorphonuclear leucocytes. All types of immune cells, including these, are found in the liver. In fact, the liver is one of the major lymphoid organs of the immune system.

The immune cells in the liver protect against infections or toxins, but may also, in certain diseases, cause liver injury. In viral hepatitis, for example, the virus alone may cause liver damage, but the inflammation caused by the immune response to the virus can produce even more damage.

Chemical Factory. Your liver acts as a chemical powerhouse—building the substances you need for life and neutralizing or safely dumping harmful material. In fact, your liver performs more than 500 complex chemical functions!

I hope you're beginning to see that your liver works overtime to help and protect you. Take your digestive system, for instance. The liver stores nutrients, then sends them out to the parts of your body that need them.

When you eat carbohydrates (potatoes, pasta, and other starches), your body breaks them down into glucose. You need glucose for energy, but because of your liver, you don't have to eat spaghetti all day long. Instead, the liver stores glucose as glycogen. When you need a burst of energy, your liver turns glycogen back into glucose and sends it through the bloodstream to your body.

Some of the fats you eat build new cells. The liver sends extra fat into the blood and, eventually, your body stores it as fat cells (adipose tissue). If you run out of carbohydrates, the fat stored in your liver becomes a major source of body fuel.

Protein you eat is broken down in your gut into amino acids, which are absorbed and distributed via the bloodstream to your liver and body. Cells use the amino acids to make new proteins or burn the amino acids for fuel. Proteins made by the liver regulate your clotting system, transport fat and nutrients throughout your body, control hormone levels, and maintain your blood volume.

Bilirubin. Bilirubin is the yellow pigment responsible for jaundice. When red blood cells in your body break down, they release hemoglobin—a molecule that carries oxygen to your tissues.

Enzymes are proteins that make specific chemical reactions take place. One of these enzymes, called heme oxygenase, occurs in bone marrow and liver cells. It converts heme, the major component of hemoglobin, into bilirubin. The liver then removes the bilirubin from your blood and turns it into a water-soluble form that is excreted into bile.

Normally, the amount of bilirubin produced approximates the rate of red blood cell breakdown. Bilirubin levels rise when something goes wrong, such as the breakdown of too many red blood cells, the development of liver disease (such as hepatitis), a defect in liver metabolism, or a blockage of the bile system. Bilirubin accumulates in tissues, causing your skin and the white part of your eyes (sclerae) to turn yellow.

ALT (SGPT), AST (SGOT), GGT, Alkaline Phosphatase. Your liver creates all of these enzymes. When liver cells are injured, the enzymes escape and enter the bloodstream. If small numbers of cells are affected, there may be little or no increase in plasma levels of enzymes. When large numbers of liver cells are injured or die, the levels of these enzymes in plasma increase markedly.

Enzyme tests roughly reflect the level of ongoing injury, but they don't indicate how your liver is actually functioning. To do that, you need to look at the tests that measure your liver's ability to build and synthesize (albumin, clotting factors) or to excrete (bilirubin).

Albumin. The liver makes this protein. It is vital for maintaining body fluid balance, especially the volume of plasma in your blood.

Although albumin levels in plasma may be affected by other disorders, in liver disease the level of serum albumin is a good marker of your liver's ability to produce proteins. A sustained decrease below the normal range is one of the first signs of advancing liver disease.

Clotting Factors. The liver also makes many proteins that help the blood to clot. In contrast to albumin, which stays a long time in plasma, clotting factors have a relatively short survival period. Therefore, the liver must constantly work to produce enough coagulation factors to maintain normal clotting.

When the liver is injured and can't make clotting factors, plasma levels drop within one or two days. Soon patients notice that they're bruising or bleeding easily even after minor bumps and injuries. If liver failure occurs, patients may hemorrhage and often require plasma and blood transfusions.

Hormones. The thyroid is one of the main hormone-producing glands. Patients with chronic hepatitis C have a high occurrence of underlying thyroid disease. Interferon therapy may cause the thyroid condition to flare. Therefore, doctors commonly run tests for thyroid function before and after interferon treatment.

In late stages of liver disease (cirrhotic phase), patients may experience other hormonal imbalances, including altered ovulation or gonadal function and impairment of the pituitary gland (the main hormone control center). For example, men with cirrhosis often develop distressing enlargement of their breasts due to hormonal imbalance. In addition, pituitary hormones regulate functions such as sleep-wake cycles, appetite, and body temperature.

My wife kept nagging me to tell the doctor how sore the nipple was on my right breast. "But what if it's cancer?" she said. At my next office visit, I worked up the nerve to ask.

"Hormones change in end-stage liver disease," my doctor said.

"Are you telling me what I think you are?"

"Yes," he said. "You're growing a breast."

I couldn't believe it. Cowboys don't grow breasts!

Larry

Phases of Hepatitis C

Figure 4B diagrams the consequences of hepatitis C infection. We divide hepatitis C infection and disease into four overlapping phases:

    I. Infection
    II. Inflammation
    III. Fibrosis
    IV. Cirrhosis

Phase I: Infection. When the hepatitis C virus gets into the bloodstream, it attaches to liver cells, enters them, and starts to reproduce. The new virus, made within the infected liver cell, exits into the bloodstream where it attaches to and infects another liver cell. This process allows the infection to spread through the liver.

Patients often ask me, "Why do I have hepatitis C if I have antibodies against hepatitis C?" Although your body produces an immune response to the virus (antibodies form and immune cells called lymphocytes are recruited into the liver), it usually doesn't get rid of the infection. We now know that approximately 85 percent of patients become chronically infected. In other infections antibodies effectively fight the infection, but in hepatitis C the antibodies are ineffective and do not clear the infection. In fact, antibodies (when present) usually indicate active disease and ongoing infection.

Phase II: Inflammation. In this phase, liver inflammation (hepatitis) develops. Under the microscope, most liver cells appear

FIGURE 4B. CONSEQUENCES OF HCV INFECTION

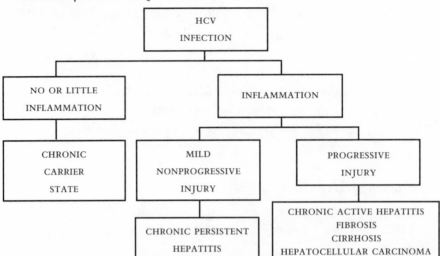

LEGEND 4B: Potential consequences of hepatitis C infection are shown. Some patients develop no or very little inflammation and co-exist with hepatitis C in a chronic carrier state. Others experience variable degrees of inflammation and liver damage. In the most severe cases, scarring becomes severe, resulting in cirrhosis or liver cancer (hepatocellular carcinoma—hepatoma).

relatively normal and uninjured. But in some areas there is liver cell injury and death. Inflammation in the liver is characterized by the presence of specific immune cells called lymphocytes. Lymphocytes are recruited to the liver to attempt to eliminate hepatitis C. However, they also release chemicals that damage liver cells and contribute to the liver injury.

In the majority of cases, the initial, acute phase of hepatitis C is mild in terms of symptoms. Most people don't realize they've had a first attack, and there are only a few cases of sudden, severe (fulminant) liver failure due to the virus. Most patients have no symptoms and only a fraction develop jaundice.

We now know that almost everyone goes on to develop chronic hepatitis. The chronic form, too, is usually mild and asymptomatic, although many patients complain of fatigue, poor stamina, and inability to concentrate.

Phase III: Fibrosis. Despite the mild nature of the inflammation and liver injury, the disease commonly progresses to fibrosis—the formation of scar tissue in the liver. If your liver biopsy shows significant fibrosis, it usually means you've had hepatitis C for more than 10 years.

Phase IV: Cirrhosis. When fibrosis increases, the fourth stage appears. With cirrhosis, the fibrosis is so severe that it affects how the liver functions and grossly distorts the architecture and blood flow of the liver.

Ten Danger Signs of Liver Disease

Warning symptoms fall into two categories: early and late. The liver sends few early warning signs. It's such a large organ with great reserve; most people can lose three-quarters of their liver without any change in function or development of symptoms.

In early hepatitis C, even though the liver is damaged, no symptoms appear. Symptoms early in the course of hepatitis C, such as muscle aches and headaches, are due to the virus itself and not to liver failure. Later in the course of hepatitis C, liver function diminishes and warning signs of advanced liver disease appear.

Early Warning Signs: #1–#2

#1: Early Symptoms. Here's Hedy:

> *At our hepatitis C support group, we compared notes. No one had serious symptoms like itching or mental confusion, even though one of us had cirrhosis. Almost everyone, however, complained of fatigue.*
>
> *It also turned out that four of us often experienced a kind of tender, achy feeling on our right sides. Doctors had dismissed the symptom by saying the liver didn't feel pain—not to worry. But of course, we did.*
>
> *So at my next medical appointment, I brought up the mystery symptom and got an answer. The liver doesn't feel pain, but the membrane around the liver and the liver itself may react to the inflammation from hepatitis.*

I reported back to the group, and we all relaxed. Nothing had changed, but the simple explanation helped. It kept us from imagining that we were sliding into liver failure.

Many people with hepatitis C, especially in the early phases, tell me they have no symptoms. I find, however, that if I question them closely, they complain of fatigue, feel less energetic, and are unable to work at their usual high level. Typically, appetite and weight are unaffected, but occasionally some patients report less enthusiasm for eating and so have difficulty maintaining their weight.

No one knows why these common symptoms occur. Some researchers think they're due to the viral infection itself, while others feel that the ongoing liver injury releases substances into the blood that produce these effects.

In my experience, these symptoms rarely, if at all, correspond to the severity of the disease. Some of my patients suffer extreme fatigue but have little injury to their livers, while others with aggressive hepatitis and cirrhosis may have no symptoms at all.

#2: Changes in Liver Functions. If you have hepatitis C, you need close medical supervision. Current recommendations call for an annual physical exam and liver blood tests every six months. Changes in blood tests usually pick up the first sign of deteriorating liver function.

Twenty-four years ago I had a really bad car accident, lost part of my liver, and had last rites. I received lots of blood transfusions. Afterwards, it was really weird. I got so tired I could barely mow my lawn.

Finally, I was diagnosed with hepatitis C. I was back in school, and right after graduation my blood tests changed. My bilirubin was up, so I was a little jaundiced. My platelet count was really low—one-third what it was supposed to be. Platelets coagulate your blood, so if I barely bumped something, my skin would tear, and I'd bleed. My nose was bleeding all the time.

Pete

At later stages of disease, albumin may decrease, bilirubin may rise, and prothrombin (a protein involved in blood clotting) time may increase. These changes occur because the liver is becoming less able to make its usual quota of substances the body needs. Another change that occurs is enlargement of the spleen. Platelets, white blood cells, and even red blood cells may drop because the enlarged spleen traps and destroys these cells. In my experience, a progressive buildup of fluid in the ankles and a low level of sodium in the blood are also common. These danger signs correlate with the cirrhotic stage. They indicate that the liver is less able to keep up with the amount of injury and often precede more serious symptoms of liver failure.

Later Warning Signs of Cirrhosis: #3–#10

What does cirrhosis mean? Cirrhosis simply means the hardening of the liver due to a buildup of scar tissue. Patients who have early-stage cirrhosis may not have any symptoms. Late stage cirrhosis is characterized by complications (some of which are life threatening) and limited survival. Patients with any or all of the following signs may be potential candidates for a liver transplant.

#3: Yellowing of the Skin and Whites of the Eyes: Jaundice. Jaundice is an accumulation of the pigment bilirubin in the skin and other tissues of the body, such as the whites of the eyes. Jaundice commonly occurs in patients with hepatitis C when the liver disease is advanced and the hepatitis flares. In some cases, jaundice may disappear when the flare resolves.

> *I was like the walking dead. My skin was a poor color—gray. Other days, I was yellow, jaundiced. I didn't think I was going to make it, but I did. The transplant worked, and I'm grateful.*
> Blaire

#4: Fluid Buildup: Ascites. Ascites means that fluid builds up in the abdomen, so that the belly swells. Liver disease is the most common cause of ascites.

I didn't realize I was holding water. I thought, "What have I eaten that's made my stomach so bloated?" At one point the doctor figured I was carrying 30 to 35 pounds of water in my stomach.

The swelling came and went, but in the last year it's been an acute problem. My fingers, knees, even my calves are swollen. My skin is so tight that my feet look like little porky pigs. The doctor gives me diuretics to make me go to the bathroom. It makes for a busy day!

Jerry

If I eat too much, the ascites gets worse. A huge meal does me in. Afterwards, I feel like I'm going to explode! The best thing is to eat in small amounts, a little bit at a time.

Josie

Physicians must remove and analyze the fluid to exclude other causes. To remove fluid the physician performs a paracentesis, which involves placing a needle through the abdominal wall and drawing out the fluid for a culture, cell count, biochemical tests, and a microscopic examination. If the ascites is due to liver disease, the fluid will be clear, yellow, uninfected, and have a low cell count.

More than one problem, however, may be involved. Sometimes patients have a bacterial infection in the ascites (spontaneous bacterial peritonitis). In these cases, there are other signs of infection: fever, high white blood count, abdominal pain. It's important to recognize this condition right away and treat it early with antibiotics. We now have many treatments for ascites, including diuretics (drugs that increase the amount of urine excreted), paracentesis (drawing off fluid), or shunts (tubes that redirect the liquid), such as peritoneovenous shunts and transjugular intrahepatic portal-systemic shunts.

Muscle cramps are a common problem in patients with advanced liver disease. In particular, patients with ascites who are treated with diuretics commonly complain of severe cramping. This type of cramping may respond to reducing diuretics or administering magnesium and calcium.

Ascites is a serious warning sign of very advanced liver disease, and most patients with ascites will require a liver transplant for prolonged survival.

#5: Bleeding: Variceal Hemorrhage. The most dramatic and urgent complication of advanced liver disease is variceal hemorrhage. "Variceal" refers to varices, which are abnormally distended or swollen veins usually located in the esophagus, and "hemorrhage," of course, means bleeding.

Patients vomit large quantities of red blood, show signs of altered mental status, and have very low blood pressure. By the time they get to the emergency room, they may be in shock.

> *I didn't know I had hepatitis C until I went into the hospital with an esophageal bleed. It was in 1991. We were having a family picnic, and I had drunk lots of cherry Kool-Aid®. I tried to convince myself the red stuff coming out of my mouth was the punch, but then I bled again. The doctors tubed me through my nose and stopped the bleeding.*
>
> *Chris*

It's urgent to get to an emergency medical facility when there's any sign of bleeding from the upper gastrointestinal tract. Variceal bleeding may be vomiting red blood, the passage of loose, dark, tarry feces, or the passage of a large amount of red blood through the rectum.

Doctors first must find the source of the bleeding before they can treat the problem. They insert a slender tube (endoscope) down the patient's throat to diagnose the cause or source of the bleed. Endoscopists have two treatments available: tying the bleeding veins with bands (ligation) or injecting a chemical into the vein to make it clot (sclerotherapy). Both therapies work well to control the initial bleed. But to eradicate the varices and avoid later hemorrhages, outpatient treatments must be repeated— usually two or three times.

Doctors may also give medications such as somatostatin, vasopressin, nitroglycerin, and plasma products to control the bleeding. Sometimes propranolol or related medicines are given to lower the risk of a rebleed.

Occasionally, varices are also found in the stomach, duodenum, intestine, and colon. It's harder to manage varices in these locations with endoscopic treatment. Doctors often will treat bleeding from these varices with either a surgical shunt (a tube that redirects the blood) or TIPS. Surgical shunts require major abdominal surgery and connect one of the portal veins to veins that bypass the liver (systemic veins).

TIPS is short for transjugular intrahepatic portal-systemic shunt. Radiologists put the TIPS in place, avoiding the need for risky abdominal surgery that might compromise a later liver transplant.

First, the radiologist places a catheter through a vein in the neck, then into the liver via the hepatic veins. A needle goes through this catheter into the liver and punctures a main branch of the portal vein. Once the portal vein and hepatic veins are connected, the radiologist dilates the tract and places an expandable cylindrical wire-mesh shunt across the liver to maintain the connection. When the shunt is in place, it relieves the back pressure on the portal veins, varices collapse, and the risk of further hemorrhage is greatly reduced.

Transplant surgeons welcome TIPS because it doesn't interfere with their surgery. However, occasionally, TIPS migrate into the portal vein and complicate a transplant operation, so most transplant doctors prefer that TIPS be placed by radiologists with a high level of experience with the procedure.

#6: Mental confusion: portal-systemic encephalopathy. The liver conducts many metabolic functions, including clearing or detoxifying the blood of harmful substances. When the liver fails, these substances may build up to toxic levels and impair the function of other organs, such as the brain.

> *Just before my liver transplant, my doctors had me take a mental test. They said there were no passing scores, and you couldn't fail—but I did. I flunked it. I know I did.*

A year after my transplant, they asked me to take it again. This time I did well. In fact, I did so well, I scored higher than a third of the doctors who took the same test!

Jack

The brain reacts to altered liver functions, so patients with advanced liver disease commonly note changes in their mental abilities. These changes range from slight changes, such as decline in memory or reduced ability to perform complex calculations, to more severe changes, such as confusion, disorientation, blackout spells, or even coma.

It helps to understand four features of encephalopathy: (1) It is usually brought on by some other problem, such as gastrointestinal bleeding, infection, or electrolyte imbalance. (2) It's a completely reversible condition. (3) Effective medical therapy exists [lactulose (a non-absorbable carbohydrate), neomycin (an antibiotic), a protein-restricted diet]. Early therapy may prevent the patient from lapsing into more advanced stages, such as coma. (4) A successful liver transplant completely reverses the condition.

This means that a patient experiencing encephalopathy must get urgent medical attention and evaluation, be treated promptly, and considered for liver transplantation.

#7: Weight Loss. Because the liver acts as your body's metabolic factory and energy storehouse, advancing liver disease affects your nutrition. That's why your doctor looks for weight loss.

I had a lot of muscle because I was a physical therapist. When I look in the mirror now, I can see the wasting. I'm so much thinner in my arms, shoulders, and back. Then again, my stomach's out to here from fluid. So I've got this weird figure.

Lila

Patients need to eat an appropriate amount of calories. And because people often are on a sodium restriction for ascites and a protein restriction for encephalopathy, that can be hard to do. I usually recommend supplements and a visit to a dietician.

Blood tests detect nutritional deficiencies. People with liver disease, for example, may have fat-soluble vitamin deficiencies (A, D, E, K) that can be at least partially corrected with oral supplements. I prefer retinyl palmitate (vitamin A), Calderol® (vitamin D-25-OH), tocopherol polyethylene glycol solution or TPGS (vitamin E), and Mephyton® (vitamin K). The TPGS formulation of vitamin E is an emulsified liquid that also aids the absorption of A, D, and K. A simple way to think of TPGS is that it's artificial bile. I recommend that all the fat-soluble vitamins be taken with the TPGS to improve absorption.

#8: Thinning of Bones (Osteoporosis) and Fractures: Metabolic Bone Disease. Did you know that as liver disease progresses, bone loss may accelerate? Bone loss is frequently observed in patients with advanced hepatitis C, especially those receiving steroid medication for other conditions.

In my whole life I had never broken any bones—pretty unusual. Then in the space of two years, I broke my toe twice. The first time, I fell off my bike; the second, I hit my toe against a floorboard. The final straw came when I fractured my kneecap. Two years later, my knee still aches when the weather changes. Coincidence, growing older, hepatitis C—who knows? But my doctor wants me to take some tests.

Sheila

First, the doctor must exclude other causes of bone loss, such as vitamin D deficiency or hyperparathyroidism. Typically, patients with bone disease and fractures due to end-stage liver disease simply have a condition called osteopenia, which does not respond well to vitamin D, calcium, or fluoride. Recent studies suggest that a new drug, alendronate, may be of some benefit. To complicate matters, post-transplant use of steroids and the relative inactivity after surgery can make the bones more brittle. Most transplant centers now taper steroids sharply and encourage early ambulation to lower the risk of fractures.

#9: Blood Clotting Problems: Coagulopathy. People with end-stage liver disease have multiple defects in their blood clotting system that put them at risk for bleeding and hemorrhage.

> *Sometimes I just bite into an apple, and I see blood right there—on the fruit. Three times in the last month I woke up with blood in my mouth.*
>
> *Also, I've been getting blood spots—like little red pimples— across my chest and arms. My wife says they look like spider veins. They don't hurt, but if I forget and scratch them, they bleed.*
>
> Gary

Coagulation proteins drop to such low levels that even minor trauma to skin, gums, lips or extremities causes marked bruising or prolonged oozing of blood. In addition, the spleen often holds and destroys platelets, reducing the body's other major clotting aid. If severe clotting disturbances develop, it's an ominous sign of advanced liver disease and means immediate consideration for a transplant.

#10: Itching: Pruritus. Although relatively uncommon in patients with hepatitis C, constant itching, day and night, may torment patients with severe jaundice or advanced liver disease. It's caused by a buildup of substances in the skin that are normally cleared by the liver, and it's not associated with hives or rashes (except what people get from scratching). Although generalized, itching may be peculiarly localized to the palms of the hands, soles of the feet, inside the mouth, and the external ear canal.

> *Excuse my language, but I call it "the bitchy itch." My symptoms began as a little itch. I hardly noticed it. I ignored it until it got bigger, and I started scratching. There was one spot the size of a quarter on my left leg. Creams did no good.*
>
> *Over a year-and-a-half it got so bad I swore I'd never scratch—and I've got high will power. But I scarred my legs.*

Finally, someone in my support group told me to use corn-starch. So now I bathe, dry myself off, and apply the cornstarch. I've done it three times so far, and it helps.

Saul

The pruritus of liver disease does not respond to antihistamines, skin lotions, and creams, but improves with the use of medicines that promote bile flow, such as ursodeoxycholate, or that bind and inactivate substances in the intestine, such as cholestyramine.

Recent studies suggest that pruritus may be related to naturally occurring morphine-like compounds that build up in the patient and may respond to medications that block morphine effects (naloxone, naltrexone).

Some patients have severe, incapacitating pruritus that can't be helped by any of the therapies mentioned. A liver transplant successfully treats the condition.

Other Related Clinical Conditions of Hepatitis C

Kidney Damage. A specific type of kidney damage, called membranoproliferative glomerulonephritis, can occur when immune complexes of the hepatitis C virus lodge in the kidney and cause inflammation. At first, there may be no symptoms. It's often detected when a routine urinalysis shows protein in the urine. As more protein is lost in urine, the blood albumin may decrease, and patients may notice swelling in the ankles or abdomen. Rarely, it can lead to kidney failure. Glomerulonephritis, complicating hepatitis C, often responds to treatment with interferon.

Cryoglobulinemia. The signs of this condition are skin rash, fever, kidney damage, and ulcerations on the fingers and toes. It's caused by antibodies that the body manufactures against the hepatitis C virus. Management of cryoglobulinemia is complex but may involve interferon, steroids, cyclophosphamide, intravenous immunoglobulins, and plasmapheresis (passing blood through a filter to remove the antibody complexes).

Thyroid Disease. Thyroid disease is very common in the

general population (2 to 3 percent) and even more common in hepatitis C patients (5 to 20 percent). Usually, it's an underactive thyroid causing the problem, but in rare cases, the thyroid can be overactive. The signs of an underactive thyroid include cold intolerance, sluggishness, dry skin, coarse hair, a change in voice, mental confusion. Signs of an overactive thyroid include palpitations, sweating, heat intolerance, jitters, tremor, poor concentrating ability, and hypertension.

An underactive thyroid is treated with thyroid hormone replacement, such as levo-thyroxine. Treatment of an overactive thyroid may involve radioactive iodine, beta-blockers, and propylthiouracil.

Skin Conditions. Skin conditions associated with hepatitis C include lichen planus, lichenoid dermatitis, and porphyria cutanea tarda. The first two are usually best treated with dermatologic lotions/creams and may flare during interferon treatment.

Lichen planus is a reddish-brown raised round spot, typically less than one to two centimeters in diameter. Sometimes it appears scaly and may itch.

Lichenoid dermatitis looks like scaly, reddish flat areas, usually larger than two centimeters in diameter. It's occasionally itchy.

Porphyria cutanea tarda appears as blisters on sun-exposed areas or areas of trauma—usually on fingers and hands. Porphyria cutanea tarda responds to iron removal by taking blood (phlebotomy) and treatment of the hepatitis C.

Autoimmune Conditions. Case reports suggest that a number of autoimmune conditions may be associated with the hepatitis C virus or interferon treatment. These include idiopathic thrombocytopenic purpura (low platelet count), autoimmune chronic active hepatitis (inflammation in the liver due to your immune system), and polyarteritis nodosa (inflammation of blood vessels—abdomen, liver, and kidney).

Disorders that may flare on interferon therapy include hemolytic anemia (red cells break down), pericarditis/pleuritis (inflammation of the lining of the heart and lung), psoriasis, rheumatoid arthritis, and systemic lupus erythematosis.

Reading this list of what can go wrong with your liver antici-pates the worst that can happen. Remember that two-thirds of the people who develop chronic hepatitis C do not progress to cir-rhosis over 20 to 30 years. Nevertheless, it's important to know what the symptoms are, so you can report any changes promptly to your physician.

In the next chapters, we'll take a look at ways you can help your liver with healthy eating habits and stress-reduction tech-niques. I'll contribute a medical perspective, we'll hear from ex-perts who specialize in these areas, and we'll listen to patients as they share their personal stories.

> *The beginning of health is to know the disease.*
>
> *Miguel de Cervantes*

References

1. Pablo Neruda. *Nuevas Odas Elementales*. Buenos Aires: Editorial Losada, p. 76-80.
2. "Sculpture in Spain Salutes the 'Silent, Unselfish' Liver," *Austin American-Statesman,* 28 June 1987:A2.

5

Taking Care of Yourself Nutritionally

Guidelines for Healthy Nutrition in Liver Disease

At first, when I was still in shock over the diagnosis of chronic hepatitis C, I was too scared to try interferon. So I decided to do all I could with "natural" methods. I went to two dieticians who recommended a low-fat diet to take a load off my liver. They also advocated intravenous vitamin C and coffee enemas, which turned me off.

Then I saw a naturopath. He restricted my diet in so many ways, I lost ten pounds. I never looked so good! But I still felt tired, so I consulted a nutritionist. She had me keep a food journal, then told me I wasn't eating enough protein. I followed her suggestions and started to feel more energy.

Looking back, I can see what I was trying to do—control what I could in a world that suddenly seemed so out of control. I might not be able to stop the virus, but I could decide what I put into my body.

After a while, I found that all the junk food I used to love didn't taste so good anymore. It seems ironic to me now, but learning I was ill made me "healthier."

Hedy

MANY PEOPLE, when they discover they have hepatitis C, become interested in improving their general health through good nutrition. I encourage patients to learn how to eat in a healthier way, but to avoid crash diets and food fads that promise more than they can deliver.

CAUTION: Always check with your doctor before making major changes in your diet or taking over-the-counter supplements and vitamins. Some seemingly harmless substances can injure your liver.

In the early, noncirrhotic stages of hepatitis C, people can maintain normal nutrition if they eat a well-balanced diet. It's rare for a doctor to recommend supplements beyond one multivitamin a day. However, as the disease progresses, malnutrition and vitamin deficiencies may develop.

Nutritional therapy includes the following goals:

• to maintain the appropriate balance between the calories you take in and the calories your body requires
• to avoid malnutrition or deficiencies in specific nutrients
• to use appropriate supplementation when needed

In this chapter, I'll discuss some general nutritional concepts, what happens when liver disease affects your nutrition, and some specific deficiencies and their treatments:

• Nutritional Overview
    Ideal Body Weight
    Normal Diet
• Nutrition and the Liver
    Carbohydrate Metabolism
    Protein Metabolism

Nutritional Overview

The liver is your body's major digestive organ. When the liver receives nutrients from the intestines, it metabolizes,* packages, stores, and sends them to other organs where they are used for energy. Your liver's major nutritional jobs include:

• metabolizing carbohydrates, proteins, and fat for energy
• assimilating and storing vitamins
• manufacturing bile to aid in digestion and absorption of fats
• filtering and destroying toxins (including alcohol and drugs)

Ideal Body Weight. Most people worry about their weight, with good reason. Many Americans weigh more than they should. With advanced liver disease, however, a major concern is the opposite problem, nutritional wasting.

What, then, should you weigh? We have no exact measure of ideal body weight because the "norm" is based on population statistics, cultural perceptions, and the influence of genetically and environmentally determined differences in metabolism. In short, there are no absolute rules, only working guidelines:

---

*Throughout this chapter we use the term "metabolism," which we define as the body processes, including a whole host of chemical reactions, that are necessary to maintain function and sustain life.

- Men: 106 pounds for the first five feet, then add six pounds for every inch thereafter
- Women: 100 pounds for the first five feet, then add five pounds for every inch thereafter

Normal Diet. Food supplies us with carbohydrates, fats, and proteins that in turn supply energy. Energy is measured in calories. Carbohydrates and proteins provide approximately four calories per gram, and fat provides almost nine calories per gram—twice as much. People also need essential nutrients (such as certain vitamins, minerals, amino acids, and fatty acids) and other substances, such as fiber, from a *variety* of foods. Oranges, for example, are rich in vitamin C, bananas supply potassium, and a half-cup serving of cantaloupe contributes half of the daily requirement for beta-carotene.

> *I was taking lots of supplements, including omega 3 oil— which tastes yucky. Then I found out that studies using fish oil supplements don't show the same results as just eating fish a couple of times a week.*
>
> *What a relief. That stuff tasted like the castor oil my mother used to dose me with every spring!*
>
> *Bonnie*

A normal, healthy diet contains the amounts of essential nutrients and calories you need to prevent either a nutritional deficiency or excess and provides the right *balance* of carbohydrate, fat, and protein. The U.S. Department of Agriculture (USDA) currently recommends a daily caloric intake of 30 to 40 calories per kilogram of body weight and the following dietary balance:

- 40 to 50 percent carbohydrate
- 30 percent fat
- 1 to 1.5 grams of protein for each kilogram (2.2 lbs.) of body weight

For more information about healthy diets, I recommend you

consult the Food Guide Pyramid published by the USDA. It graphically illustrates the importance of balance among different food groups in a daily eating pattern and suggests the number (depending on daily calorie intake desired) and size of daily servings.

Serving sizes are small. For example, one serving equals one-half cup of pasta; one cup of raw, leafy vegetables; one-half cup of other vegetables (cooked or chopped raw); one medium apple, banana, orange; one cup of milk or yoghurt; or two to three ounces of cooked lean meat, poultry, or fish.

The USDA recommendations include a range of servings from each of the five major food groups. People who consume about 1,600 calories a day should be guided by the smaller number; the larger number is for people who are very active and consume about 2,800 calories a day:

- Choose most of your daily foods from the bread, cereal, rice, and pasta group (6–11 servings), vegetable group (3–5 servings), and fruit group (2–4 servings).
- Choose moderate amounts of foods from the milk, yoghurt, and cheese group (2–3 servings) and the meat, poultry, fish, dry beans, eggs, and nuts group (2–3 servings).
- Limit foods that provide few nutrients and are high in fat and sugar.
- In general, the USDA recommends a diet moderate in salt and sodium and low in fat, saturated fat, and cholesterol.

Resource: For a free copy of *Dietary Guidelines for Americans*, U.S. Department of Agriculture, call the USDA Center for Nutrition Policy and Promotion Publication Line: 202-606-8000. You may also request additional information on nutrition from the Center by writing to them at the following address: 1120 20th St., NW, Suite 200, North Lobby, Washington, DC 20036.

Resource: The American Dietetic Association's National Referral Line (for qualified dieticians in your area) is 1-800-366-1655.

Resource: The American Institute for Cancer Research provides practical tips on good nutrition with its newsletter, pamphlets, and a toll-free AICR Nutrition Hotline staffed by a registered dietician: Call 1-800-843-8114 and ask for Nutrition Information.

Nutrition and the Liver

The liver is the major organ responsible for regulating and responding to your body's metabolic demands. Your liver must be functioning well to maintain normal metabolism of carbohydrates, fats, and protein; it is also responsible for processing and using several vitamins. This section deals with the role a healthy liver (and a healthy, well-balanced diet) plays in these nutritional processes.

Carbohydrate Metabolism. The most common sources of dietary carbohydrate are sugars, such as sucrose (table sugar), fructose (corn syrup), and lactose (milk sugar), and starches, such as breads, pasta, grains, cereals, fruits, vegetables, and potatoes. When you eat carbohydrates, specialized enzymes in the pancreas and gut process them to yield simple sugars (glucose, galactose, fructose, maltose).

These sugars are absorbed by intestinal lining cells, enter the portal circulation, and travel to the liver via the portal vein. During overnight fasting, blood sugar levels dip to a relatively low level, insulin secretion is suppressed, and blood insulin levels diminish. After a meal, blood sugar increases (stimulating the release of insulin from the pancreas), and insulin levels rise. Insulin, which rises in response to a meal, is the hormone that stimulates the liver to take in more glucose and to move the glucose into storage—mainly in the form of glycogen. The liver can then release glycogen to your muscles for energy during periods of fasting or exercise. Although the liver can store considerable amounts of glycogen, it is the first energy source used during periods of prolonged fasting or caloric deprivation, and it can be depleted rapidly. After glycogen, the body taps other energy sources—including protein and fat.

Protein Metabolism. We take in dietary protein from dairy products, produce, and meats. Enzymes produced by the pancreas and intestine break down the protein into its amino acids and small peptides. The intestine rapidly absorbs the amino acids with

TABLE 5A. SOME COMMON LIVER PROTEINS AND
THEIR FUNCTION IN THE HUMAN BODY

Protein	Function
Clotting factors (II, V, VII, IX, and X)	Maintain normal clotting
Albumin	Maintain normal blood volume
Renin	Regulate blood pressure
Binding globulins	Regulate hormone action
Transferrin	Transport iron
Ferritin	Store iron
Retinol binding protein	Transport vitamin A to the eye
LDL receptor	Remove cholesterol from the blood
P-450 proteins	Metabolize drugs, chemicals, toxins

specific transport systems within its lining cells and then delivers the amino acids to the liver via the portal vein.

When they reach the liver, they are used for energy or for making (synthesizing) new proteins. The newly synthesized proteins perform specific body functions (see Table 5A).

Fat Metabolism. In general, fats are neutral lipids (triglycerides), acidic lipids (fatty acids), and sterols (cholesterol, plant sterols). Triglycerides (dairy products, meats, oils, butter, margarine) are the most common type of dietary fat and represent a major source of energy. The liver is uniquely suited to regulate and process triglycerides.

Dietary triglyceride is digested in the intestine by lipase, an enzyme secreted by the pancreas in response to meals. Bile, secreted by the liver, makes the digested fat soluble and promotes its absorption. Absorbed fat is then repackaged and transported into blood, where the liver ultimately removes it from the circulation. Fat that reaches the liver is processed in three ways: (1) stored as fat droplets in liver cells, (2) metabolized as a source of energy, and (3) repackaged, secreted back into blood, and delivered to other cells in the body.

The liver is also intimately involved with the processing of dietary cholesterol and is the main source of newly synthesized cholesterol in the body. Liver disease may be associated with both high or low blood cholesterol levels. In general, as liver disease progresses in patients with hepatitis C, the blood level of cholesterol drops.

Bile. The liver produces and secretes a fluid (bile) that enters the intestine to aid in digestion and absorption. Bile is clear yellow to golden-brown and contains water, electrolytes (salts), cholesterol, bile salts (detergents), phospholipids, and proteins. Bile helps to activate enzymes secreted by the pancreas and is essential for the digestion and absorption of fat or fat-soluble vitamins.

Vitamins. The liver plays a role in several steps of vitamin metabolism. I'll describe only a few of those steps. Vitamins are either fat-soluble (Vitamins A, D, E, and K) or water-soluble (Vitamin C and the B-complex vitamins).

Patients with advanced liver disease may become deficient in water-soluble vitamins, but this is usually due to inadequate nutrition and poor food intake. Vitamin B_{12} storage usually far exceeds the body's requirements; deficiencies rarely occur due to liver disease or liver failure. When dietary intake drops, however, thiamine and folate commonly become deficient. Oral supplementation is usually all that you need to restore thiamine and folate stores to the normal range.

Fat-soluble vitamins require not only adequate dietary intake but also good digestion and absorption by the body. That's why normal production of bile is essential. Bile in the gut is required for the absorption of fat-soluble vitamins into the body because these vitamins are relatively insoluble in water. Bile acts as a detergent, breaking down and dissolving these vitamins so they may be properly absorbed.

If bile production is poor, oral supplementation of vitamins A, D, E, and K may not be sufficient to restore vitamin levels to normal. The use of a detergent-like solution of liquid vitamin E (TPGS) improves the absorption of vitamin E in patients with advanced liver disease. The same solution may also improve the absorption of vitamins A, D, and K if the latter are taken simultaneously with the liquid vitamin E.

Nutritional Needs for Hepatitis C Patients Who Don't Have Cirrhosis

Caloric Requirements. In general, the noncirrhotic patient with hepatitis C has caloric needs similar to those of noninfected people of the same age and gender. For this reason we recommend the following:

- no salt restriction
- no protein restriction
- 30 to 40 calories per kilogram intake per day
- one multivitamin per day

Patients who drink excessive amounts of alcohol should stop drinking altogether. They may also need supplementation with thiamine and folate.

Vitamin Supplements. In general, noncirrhotic patients with hepatitis C do not require any additional vitamin supplementation other than that noted above. One concern is that if bile production drops, the patient may become deficient in fat-soluble vitamins during the course of hepatitis C infection. This deficiency rarely develops during the early stages of hepatitis C, but it may be fairly prevalent at later, cirrhotic stages of the disease. When detected, deficiencies of fat-soluble vitamins should be corrected by administering proper doses of the compounds.

Nutritional Therapies. Americans spend some $6 billion annually on nutritional supplements. Patients with viral hepatitis have used a number of such "nutritional supplements," such as echinaceae, pycnogenol, dandelion root, silymarin (milk thistle), and a wide array of herbal remedies. None of these have been studied in controlled trials and, thus, are unproved therapies.

Despite the lack of supporting data, the use of these therapies has gained widespread acceptance among patients with hepatitis C. Several factors seem to account for this phenomenon: a history of lack of effective therapies for liver disease in general; incompletely effective treatment for hepatitis C; a general attitude that, "It can't hurt me, and maybe it'll help"; and the relatively mild and slowly progressive nature of hepatitis C. However, because proof of their effectiveness is lacking, we cannot endorse or recommend that patients undergo nutritional therapies. You should, however, inform your doctor if you are considering taking any of these nutritional supplements.

> I went to a health food store and asked them to give me anything that would help my liver. I got coltsfoot, comfrey, petasites, chaparral, and yohimbe.
>
> My enzymes shot up to 800. When the doctor asked me if I was taking anything new, I brought in the bottles and learned that these herbs were best avoided because they may be toxic for the liver. I stopped taking them, and my enzymes went back down. I never thought anything "natural" could harm me.
>
> *Harold*

Nutrition Tips from Patients

People with hepatitis C who are interested in nutrition find many ways to work toward healthier eating habits. Here are some of their suggestions:

> I think you're crazy if you have hepatitis C and you drink alcohol. It's like taking poison.
>
> *Annie*

> I try to be kind to my liver. I've switched to eating more complex carbohydrates, like veggies, fruits, whole grains. If Olympic athletes train on complex carbs for energy, I guess it's good for me, too.
>
> *Shawn*

> I've given up caffeine. I figure it can't do my liver any good. So every morning I have hot water with a bit of fresh lemon in it. It was hard to switch at first, but I'm used to it now.
>
> *Dana*

I don't tolerate fats as well as I did. I can't handle the beans, chili, and tortillas I used to eat—too fatty and salty. I can't handle fried foods at all. When I cook at home, I use mostly olive oil—sometimes canola oil.

Casey

Eating small meals several times a day works better for me than eating a few large meals because I don't have much appetite. I also keep unsalted nuts in the car, in case I need a quick protein snack.

Rita

Hot oatmeal tastes good on a cold morning. To add a little protein, I sprinkle some unsalted nuts on top. Also—to avoid using too much sugar, I add just a little bit of maple syrup. It's sugar, too, but a little goes a long way.

Mindy

I used to drink 2 percent milk. Turns out that it is not low in fat. In fact, 35 percent of its calories comes from fat. So I switched to skim milk. Now I like it just as well, and it has almost no fat in it.

I used to drink lots of soda, too, until I looked at the labels— lots of sugar and salt and preservatives. I stopped all soda about a year ago. The other day I took a taste of a friend's drink and almost spit it out. My taste buds have changed.

Jason

You should see my new juicer. I'm a little intimidated by it, but I made the sweetest, freshest tasting carrot juice today. I've also heard that a carrot, beet, and cucumber combo is good, too. I figured I'd drink some of my veggies.

Brenda

A lot is attitude. If you think of a healthy, low-fat diet as a pleasure—not a burden—you can get into it. I take the time to

*shop in a really pleasant supermarket or health food store, and I
try to add new fruits and vegetables to my meals or snacks.*

*I try to sit down and not eat on the run. My biggest problem
is that I have to eat out a lot for business, but I've learned to order fish and rice more often.*

Stacey

Nutritional Needs for Hepatitis C Patients with Cirrhosis

Caloric Requirements. In general, the patient with early-stage
or compensated cirrhosis still requires 30 to 40 calories per kilogram a day. You may need to alter your dietary habits to take in
this number of calories, because as hepatitis C progresses to cirrhosis, you may begin to experience loss of appetite, increasing
fatigue, reduction in physical activity, and alteration of your sleep-
wake pattern. People commonly complain of loss of exercise tol-
erance ("I'm just too pooped out to get my work done"). In
addition, these changes often precipitate a sense of despondency,
anxiety, or depression. It helps to develop both a pattern of meals
that allows you to use your diet for maximum energy and a rest
pattern that reduces prolonged periods of physical activity.

No nutritional prescription is right for every patient. You need
to address your specific nutritional needs with your physician. In
my experience, patients with hepatitis C who develop compensated cirrhosis benefit by more frequent, smaller volume meals. Instead of one or two large meals, divide the equivalent amount of
calories into four smaller meals. In addition, supplementation with
one or two tablets of multivitamins is generally indicated, although
the overall benefit is unclear. Despite this change in dietary habit,
fatigue often persists. People benefit from "rest periods," usually
30 minutes or an hour in the mid-afternoon.

CAUTION: Please understand that advanced cirrhosis is associated with severe impairment of liver function and that specific
dietary modifications may be necessary and could alter the general
guidelines noted above. Your doctor may recommend a consulta-

tion with a dietician or provide you with a specific nutritional prescription.

Protein Restriction. It is important that the patient with cirrhosis take in enough protein to avoid excessive muscle wasting and energy depletion. However, if encephalopathy develops, a doctor might prescribe a "protein-restricted" diet.

Encephalopathy is the alteration or cloudiness of mental function. When the condition is severe, the patient becomes disoriented, confused, combative, or even comatose. Encephalopathy may also cause altered sleep-wake patterns, altered personality, and lack of motor coordination.

One factor contributing to these symptoms is dietary protein intake, so patients with any of the above symptoms may be placed on protein restrictions. This diet is usually not zero protein, but a reduced level of 20 to 60 grams per day. Often, the physician will use other treatments in conjunction with this diet, such as lactulose or neomycin.

> *While I was waiting for my liver transplant, I'd get in the car and forget if I was leaving or coming. If you've got too much protein, it can cause you to fall asleep at the intersection. The doctor told me to stop driving and put me on a protein-restricted diet. I watch the amount I take in, and if I feel too tired, I cut back. It took lots of modification to eat more vegetables. I eat them like medicine, but I'm getting better at it.*
>
> *I'm from South Dakota. I was raised on meat and potatoes. In fact, my parents joke that I was 16 before I found out that gravy wasn't a beverage!*
>
> *Bill*

Vitamin Supplements. Most people with hepatitis C, even those with cirrhosis, have adequate intake and storage of water-soluble vitamins (C, B complex). To be sure, I recommend the addition of two tablets of multivitamins each day (one in the morning and one in the evening).

Patients who excessively use or abuse alcohol risk becoming

deficient in these vitamins, particularly thiamine and folate, and they may benefit from taking supplements. As I have emphasized before, the hepatitis C patient should avoid alcohol. Those who avoid alcohol probably won't require either supplement.

There are few data on the overall extent of vitamin deficiencies in patients with hepatitis C. However, as part of our evaluation of cirrhotic patients for liver transplantation, we assessed the plasma levels of certain vitamins and found that approximately 20 percent of hepatitis C patients were deficient in vitamin A, vitamin D (25-OH), and vitamin E. Although few patients had symptoms that could be attributed to these deficiencies, it seems reasonable to monitor patients' vitamin levels as cirrhosis progresses and give supplements to those with low levels.

Mineral Supplements. Patients with cirrhosis may experience deficiencies in three minerals: calcium, magnesium, and zinc. Calcium deficiency may be related to a lack of vitamin D, poor nutrition, or malabsorption. Correcting the underlying abnormality may be all that is required to restore calcium balance. However, bone thinning may occur even without these specific problems, so I recommend 0.5 to 1.0 grams of calcium each day. Calcium may be taken in the form of dairy products or therapeutic supplements. When the patient can't take in enough dairy products because of protein, salt, or fluid restrictions (see next section), supplements are used.

Magnesium deficiency may occur due to inadequate dietary intake. However, it occurs more often when patients take diuretics to treat fluid retention because their kidneys flush out the magnesium as waste. Symptoms of magnesium deficiency include muscle cramps, fatigue, weakness, nausea, and vomiting. Often, it's not possible to modify or discontinue diuretics in cirrhotic patients, so magnesium supplementation (500 mg. magnesium gluconate three times a day) may be required.

Zinc deficiency may cause the loss of the senses of smell and taste. Patients with these symptoms may benefit from supplementation with zinc sulfate (220 mg. three times a day).

Salt and Fluid Restriction. Cirrhosis disturbs the regulation of body salt and water. Severe liver disease generates neural and hormonal signals to the kidney that cause the kidney to retain both salt and water. The salt acts like a sponge. As a result, fluid accumulates in certain tissues and body spaces, such as the ankles (peripheral edema), abdomen (ascites), and chest (pleural effusion).

> *The dietician restricted me to 2,000 milligrams of sodium a day. That's one teaspoon! I try, but I really like salt. If I don't watch carefully, though—say I eat some broth, and it has salt in it—I pick up extra water. It takes days to flush it out.*
>
> *I can get 11 to 14 pounds of fluid out every few days. Once I had 30 pounds of water on me. I had a belly like a pregnant rhino.*
>
> *My wife says if I wouldn't cover everything with "white death," I'd do a lot better.*
>
> *Randy*

Treatment of fluid retention always requires dietary salt restriction, often requires diuretics (medicines that block the kidney and cause increased urination of salt and water), and sometimes requires fluid restriction. Patients need to understand that the major driving force behind the accumulation of fluid is the excessive retention of salt. Diuretics work because they cause the kidney to lose salt. If you take in too much salt in your diet, you'll cause more fluid to accumulate in your body. In other words, you can override the effects of the diuretics, and patients on diuretics can actually retain fluid if they don't comply with a salt-restricted diet.

The usual salt restriction is two grams per day (see Table 5B). Commonly used diuretics are Aldactone® (spironolactone), Midamor® (amiloride), Lasix® (furosemide), HCTZ® (hydrochlorothiazide), and Zaroxylyn® (metolozone). Aldactone® and Midamor® conserve potassium, while Lasix®, HCTZ®, and Zaroxylyn® waste potassium. Most of the time, a doctor will prescribe the two types of diuretics together to minimize any changes in blood potassium levels. Occasionally, potassium supplements are used to keep blood potassium in the normal range.

TABLE 5B. 2-GRAM SALT DIET SAMPLE MENU★

Breakfast (352–765 mg)
  1–2 pieces toast (150–400 mg)
  1–2 tsp. margarine (50 mg)
  1 Tbs. orange marmalade
  1 boiled egg (62 mg)
        or 1 fried egg (162 mg)
  1 C cooked cereal with little or no salt (1 mg)
  ½–1 C milk (60–120 mg)
  6 oz. brewed coffee (4 mg)/tea (5 mg)/herbal tea (2 mg)
  1 C cantaloupe (14 mg) or strawberries (2 mg)
  1 C orange juice (2 mg)

Lunch (503–611 mg)
  3.5 oz. salmon patty (96 mg)
  1 slice tomato (½ mg) and ½ C lettuce (1 mg)
  1 oz. potato chips (about 10 chips) (170 mg)
  1 C fresh grapes (2 mg)
  1 C apple juice (7 mg)
  1 carrot (25 mg) and 1 stalk of celery (35 mg)
  1 piece angel food cake [161 mg (homemade); approx. 270 mg (pack-aged mix)]
  8 oz. ice tea (5 mg) with lemon (less than 1 mg)

Dinner (431–601 mg)
  3.5 oz. roast beef (63–73 mg) au jus with no added salt (if packaged
        gravy mix, 2 oz. = approx. 160 mg)
  1 baked potato (16 mg)
  1 Tbsp. sour cream (6 mg)/margarine (100 mg)
  ½ C frozen green beans (3 mg)
  1½ C tossed fresh salad (5 mg) with salt-free salad dressing
  1 piece apple pie (181 mg) with ½ C vanilla ice cream (53 mg)
  6 oz. coffee (4 mg)

★*Sodium levels generally refer to fresh homemade items, are approximate, and vary with brand names of products used. Fast, pre-packaged, or canned foods usually contain much higher levels of sodium.*

The physician usually orders fluid restriction only for edematous patients with low levels of sodium in their blood. Fluid restriction means restriction of all fluids: water, tea, coffee, milk, etc. Patients with severe symptomatic low blood sodium may find it necessary to restrict their fluid intake to less than one quart a day.

CAUTION: Always consult with your physician regarding use of diuretics (doses and frequency) or dietary restrictions on salt or fluid intake. It is potentially dangerous to self-medicate or introduce dietary restrictions without physician consultation.

He who keeps on eating after his stomach is full
digs his grave with his teeth.

Turkish proverb

6

Taking Care of Yourself Emotionally

Emotional Challenges of Chronic Illness

As a person with hepatitis C, I live with the emotional highs and lows of this disease. Every blood test and biopsy report shakes me up. Every time I get tired and can't get through a job that I used to do easily, I get angry and discouraged. It's a struggle not to get obsessed with my health.

Some days, I get mad when my friends act too protective, and other times I get mad when they leave me alone. It's hard to shake off the sadness. And then there are those glorious moments—a crisp fall day, a family dinner—when life is a gift that's unbearably beautiful.

In this chapter, Dr. Everson and I draw on the expertise of mental health professionals who work with hepatitis C patients. We also present the experiences of the patients themselves. Who else really understands?

Hedy

Here are the topics we'll cover:

- The Emotional Challenge
- Phase 1: Diagnosis
    Special Problems with a Diagnosis of Hepatitis C
- Phase 2: Impact (Attitudes and Expectations)
- Phase 3: Reorganization
- Healing vs. Curing
- Warning Signs of Depression
- Understanding your Family and Friends (Family Systems)
    Boundaries
- Tools for Wellness: Some Practical Suggestions
    Medical Care and Psychological Help
    Exercise and Nutrition
    Feeling Useful/Having Fun
    Exploring Your Creative and Spiritual Sides

HEPATITIS C may be the biggest emotional challenge you'll ever face. How do you deal with chronic disease without letting it take over your life?

"The goal is balance," says Meredith Pate-Willig, a licensed clinical social worker. Ms. Pate-Willig facilitates support groups for Colorado's The Hep C Connection and Qualife, an organization that seeks to enrich the quality of life for people facing life-challenging illness.

How do you achieve balance and a "wellness lifestyle?" "There's no short cut through normal, natural cycles of grief," says Pate-Willig. "Grieving is nature's way of helping us adapt to new information about our illness."

Too often, we're hard on ourselves as we grieve. In a world of instant cereal and microwave popcorn, we think we should be grieving faster, better. The truth is, each one of us goes through the process in our own time frame and in our own way—and the healing ingredient is kindness. Be patient with yourself. You will work it through, and you will come out of the crisis with a stronger sense of who you are.

According to Pate-Willig, it's helpful to think of these spiraling cycles of grief in three phases: diagnosis, impact, and reorganization.

Phase 1: Diagnosis

Diagnosis plunges you into a state of disbelief or shock.

> *I didn't realize it then, but it was the day my life changed forever. I was numb. I didn't even know that I was feeling shock and grief at what I had lost—my sense of health. When I walked out to the parking lot, the sun was still shining, but everything looked different. It felt unreal.*
>
> Dave

If you lose your sense of yourself as a healthy person, and you struggle or rebel against becoming a patient, how do you adjust? Some patients develop a sense of grief. Grieving is one way we work through loss, whether it's loss of our old selves ("I used to cook big family dinners. Now I'm too tired.") or loss of our dreams ("Will I ever marry now? Know my grandchildren? Launch a new business?"). According to Pate-Willig, "Grieving is normal—even necessary. It's the bridge between what was to what is. If you don't go across that bridge, you may face a continuing struggle."

In this first phase of diagnosis, you need your family and support system to pull together to help you adjust:

1. The diagnosis may make you feel uncomfortable or leave you with a numbing sense of shock and loss. You should understand that this response is normal.
2. Everyone needs psychological and social support—not just the person with hepatitis C. Other family members may be affected by the diagnosis. When one part of a system changes, everything in the system reacts in a "ripple" effect.

> *When I was first diagnosed, I went numb. The first person I told was my best friend. She broke down—a flood of tears. I was*

*horrified to find that my inner reaction was rage. I wanted to yell,
"Hey, just a minute. I'm the one with the problem here!"*

*Thank goodness, I didn't say anything out loud, but I was
mad until I realized that she had her own grief about losing me,
her best friend, as she's always known me. Her world was shaken
up, too.*

*All I wanted, all I ever really want even now, is for someone
to put an arm around me and say, "I'm here. I know this is hard.
I care about you."*

Estelle

People may not respond to you in the way that you anticipate
or expect. You may process the information fast while family
members take longer, or the reverse. How fast or how slowly
people absorb the news affects the dynamics in a marriage or
friendship—leaving everyone with the unconscious feeling that
somehow the rules changed. In fact, just identifying these changes
takes a while.

Sometimes, the patient or support system refuses to accept the
new reality. "Denial," says Pate-Willig, "is a misunderstood defense. When it acts as a circuit-breaker, it keeps your system from
overloading. That can be healthy. Denial becomes unhealthy
when it keeps you from finding appropriate medical treatment."

Special Problems with a Diagnosis of Hepatitis C

Dealing with a diagnosis of any chronic illness is difficult, but patients with hepatitis C have special issues:

Feeling Low. You may be experiencing fatigue, low energy,
loss of ability to concentrate, and a sense of inadequacy in doing
daily tasks. These symptoms may make you more emotionally
vulnerable and susceptible to periods of depression. Be sure to tell
your doctor if you feel seriously depressed.

Feeling Contaminated. Although the virus is transmitted
only by blood-to-blood contact, you may have questions and
fears about who will avoid you. How will your friends or boss react? What do you tell your dentist?

I can't believe this guy at work. I left a can of pop on the table for a minute, and he drank it by mistake. He freaked out when he found out it was mine. Now he won't even talk to me if he can help it. When he passes my desk, he won't even look me in the eye!

Bonnie

How You Got Infected. When you try to figure out how this happened to you, your answer may affect how you deal with your diagnosis: (1) If you can point to a blood transfusion, you don't feel responsible for your illness; (2) if you've injected drugs, whether it was a minor episode or you're still involved, you have to process the painful idea that you did this to yourself; (3) people who don't know how they got infected may never figure it out, and that uncertainty creates its own dilemmas.

Looking Good. Strange as it sounds, people often have trouble offering comfort to someone who doesn't have a visible wound. In the early and middle stages of infection, you may suffer silent symptoms, such as fatigue and joint pains. Unfortunately, many people (including yourself) may have a hard time believing you're ill. Unless you explain the nature of hepatitis C, you may not get the support you need.

For years before I was diagnosed, I dealt with an energy level that seemed to be going downhill. I stopped playing tennis because I couldn't run fast enough to get to the ball. I had to give up biking when my knees ached so bad.

Now I just learned I have hepatitis C, but my wife doesn't listen. "You look fine," she says. "You're just getting older."

George

Fluctuating Nature of Hepatitis C. Who knows why Jill's PCR assay shows a low viral load one month but a sky-high count the next? The fluctuating course of hepatitis C sometimes gives the patient the feeling of walking on shifting sand, never knowing what each day will bring.

Lack of Information. Uncertainty due to lack of information is a huge stressor. You have no way to answer the questions, "What am I dealing with, and how will it affect my life?" What facts your doctor offers you about your stage of illness, therefore, have a big influence on how you deal with the diagnosis.

What Can You Do to Help Yourself? "Be patient with yourself," says Pate-Willig. "Accept that this is a difficult time, and try not to beat yourself up for being normal, human."

> *The results of my second biopsy sent me into a tailspin. My liver was worse! It was like going back to the first day I was told I had hepatitis C. For days and weeks I struggled to control panic attacks and crying jags. I couldn't get on top of it.*
>
> *Finally, a friend with hepatitis C told me not to stuff the pain and sadness. "The only thing that works for me," she said, "is to feel it all the way."*
>
> *When I gave myself time to feel whatever it was—no matter how painful—I was able to move on with the rest of my day. I didn't get stuck.*
>
> *Lanie*

"Remember to be kind to yourself. Patience, patience, and more patience. That's the key," says Pate-Willig. "Expect to feel emotional cycles, ups and downs, each time the activity of your disease changes or you experience a new symptom."

Phase 2:
Impact (Attitudes and Expectations)

In Phase 1, the task for you and your support system is to pull together to confront and understand the new diagnosis. In the second phase, the question becomes, "How do we function now that we know that hepatitis C is a chronic condition? How do we gear up for the long haul?" It's a time of changing attitudes and expectations as you explore your options.

The challenge is how to connect with friends and family and

still maintain the autonomy and space you need. Your questions may vary from large ("I'm a single parent with no one to care for me. Should I go back to my mom and dad's house or keep my own apartment?") to small ("My husband had a transplant. Should I play in my Thursday night bowling league or stay home with him?").

Families often have unspoken rules and myths about illness. Perhaps the message you got was, "Keep a stiff upper lip and don't show you're scared." Or maybe you grew up in a home where a cold meant deluxe pampering. What happens if you break these rules?

> *I finally told my older brother how scared and panicky I felt. It turned out that my brother had a friend who also had hepatitis C. "He doesn't make any big deal," my brother said. "In fact, he won't even discuss it. He believes in a positive outlook."*
>
> *Compared to my brother's friend, I was a big complainer. Of course, that was my secret fear all along—being the family wimp.*
>
> *Melissa*

Phase 3: Reorganization

As you move into Phase 3, you and your family begin to reorganize around the new reality. A sense of acceptance emerges, and you start to answer these questions: Who am I now? How am I going to make my life work?

At some point, things settle down. Perhaps you come to terms with a reduced energy level, make dietary changes, decide on a treatment plan.

> *It got to be too much for me. I couldn't even cope with a full work day. Cassie and I had planned a mountain climbing vacation in the Rockies, but we decided to spend a week at a bed and breakfast with a mountain view instead. Finally, I had to accept reality.*
>
> *Jim*

Anything that tips the precarious balancing act shakes the system. If you start interferon treatment, you and your family and friends may need to organize around the treatment. Suppose you decide to plan a nap each day, while someone else assumes your chores. What most people don't realize is that *any* change, positive or negative, alters the system. So, paradoxically, you may need to reorganize after you have finished interferon treatment. For example, you may still feel the need for a daily nap, but the people around you may now disapprove.

The cycle of confronting the diagnosis, feeling its impact, and reorganizing yourself to deal with hepatitis C may recur with each piece of health news. If hepatitis C moves into advanced liver disease and a possible transplant, the concept of death may come to the forefront.

"The first big breakthrough for most people is the realization of how physically fragile we humans are," says Pate-Willig. "It's a difficult task to process, reprioritize, accept your mortality, and—at the same time—plan for post-transplant living."

Healing vs. Curing

"We are all desperate for curing," says Pate-Willig, "but a physical cure may be years away. We need to shift to healing—a balance and wholeness of mind, body, and spirit.

"As we become more aware of our emotional responses, we learn how healthy it is to *lean* into the grief process and accept it. We learn how to tap into resources that can help, such as dietary changes and relaxation techniques. The goal is to come out of each cycle at a higher level, to feel better about ourselves, and to see more flexibility in ourselves and others as we learn how to cope."

Grief can be the great healer. Grief is to the psyche and the spirit what the physical process is to the healing of a wound.

So, you say, "That sounds great. But how do I grieve?"

"Talk about what's happening to you," says Pate-Willig. Talk to a friend, a support group, a journal. Get on the Internet. Help yourself by re-evaluating your feelings each time you tell and retell your story. As you do this, you fit your new self into your old idea of yourself.

"The Chinese symbol for crisis is both danger and opportunity. Chronic illness can give us the opportunity to become deeper, broader, more flexible, and to find meaning in our lives."

Warning Signs of Depression

While grieving and depression are normal, sustained depression is not. Fortunately, there are many ways to treat depression with medications and "talk" therapy, so it's important to tell your doctor, advises Robert House, M.D., Director of Residency Training and the Department of Psychiatric Consultation Liaison Service for the University of Colorado Health Sciences Center.

What are the signs of depression? According to Dr. House, be on the alert for some of these symptoms, if they are *changes* from your normal behavior pattern:

- low energy, fatigue, lack of interest in your usual activities
- withdrawn and/or irritable behavior
- sleep disturbances that show a change in your routine pattern (such as sleeping less or more, waking up a lot, or waking earlier or later than usual, not rested and ready to begin the day)
- significant weight loss over a short period of time
- loss of appetite, food doesn't taste good
- tearfulness, breaking into tears for no apparent reason, "out of the blue"
- forming and talking about ideas of suicide, or a sense that life is not worth living
- feeling of hopelessness, helplessness that things won't get better
- reluctance to resume activities of daily living after a transplant (such as not getting along with your family, if you've always done so before; not resuming sexual relations with your spouse after a reasonable length of time; not dating, if single; isolating yourself from others)

Understanding Your Family and Friends (Family Systems)

Chronic illness is a family illness. When one member of a family becomes sick, it affects everyone. Normally, a family stays in balance with its own set of unwritten roles and rules. Roles involve position (Who is the breadwinner? Who takes out the garbage?). Roles always change as the patient needs to do less and shifts tasks to others. Rules are values; they can be about communication (Who can say what to whom?), emotion (Who is allowed to be sad?), education, sex, religion, and parenting.

Most important for people with hepatitis C are the family rules and values about health and illness. Problems arise when your family rules (or the rules of the family you grew up in) clash. Can you take time off if you have a cold or only if you're deathly ill? How do you handle the medical system?

My husband and I are having a hard time about my hepatitis C. He's an exercise nut and overdoses on vitamins. I do what my doctor tells me, and that's enough. My husband is constantly after me to change my lifestyle, and I get exasperated. I want to shout at him, "Leave me alone. I'll do it my way!"

Janice

Boundaries. Families create different boundaries. Some are so enmeshed that it's hard to tell where one member begins and another ends. They know how to pull together but need to learn how to allow outsiders to help. At the other end of the spectrum is the disengaged family where members have a high degree of autonomy and very little strong communication with each other. They need to learn how to draw closer together, so they can hear each other and support one another. Most families, of course, fall somewhere in between these two extremes.

My sister would say, "Come on, let's go shopping." I didn't want to go because the interferon treatment made me tired. I knew she'd get mad if I had to leave in a couple of hours. So I'd say no. Then she'd glare at me and preach to me. She was always trying to control me.

We had a blowout. We had been inseparable, and suddenly we weren't speaking.

Sally

Chronic illness can cause disorganization, but this crisis can open more options and choices as the family modifies and changes its rules and values.

My mom always said it was hard to believe someone was sick unless you could see a bleeding wound. But she stuck up for me all through my interferon treatment. Even though she's 85, and you'd think it would be hard for her to change, she was—and still is—the one person who understands what I'm going through.

Pete

Families also go through life stages that have their own issues of separateness and connectedness, from the birth of a child to taking care of elderly parents. When illness occurs, it can disrupt the normal tasks of these life stages. Suppose, for example, that hepatitis C strikes a parent of a teenager. The teenager will feel pulled by conflicting forces: the need to separate and develop a life with peers versus the need to pull closer to the family. In this setting the adolescent must cope with developing separateness and freedom and providing more help with household or other chores.

Communication and openness are the keys to improving the level of understanding within your family. When family members talk about a problem in terms of shifts in roles, rules and life stages, it diffuses the personal element. Usually, people feel hurt when a conflict arises because they think the other family members don't care about them. When you define the problem as a conflict in family roles, values, or degree of separation/connection, you can work toward a resolution.

Suppose, for example, that George wants his wife, Susan, to come with him to all his medical appointments. Meanwhile, Susan has had to take a part-time job to help pay the bills. Even though it's no one's fault, she's angry. Susan can't do it all, and her former role as the family's primary emotional support needs to be modified. Instead of blaming each other and feeling unloved, Susan and George talk about the role changes and come up with a compromise. Susan will go to the important medical appointments, and George will ask his sister to accompany him to the routine ones.

Do people want to change a family system? No, but illness brings unavoidable changes and, therefore, a feeling of loss of control. You can choose to be angry, or you can decide what can be changed and what cannot. How can we figure out a new system that's fair to everybody? What roles and values can we let go or modify?

Tools for Wellness: Some Practical Suggestions

Life-challenging illnesses, like hepatitis C, present opportunities for re-thinking priorities. We may not always be able to cure the disease, but we can improve the quality of our lives. We can nourish ourselves by getting good medical and psychological care, exercising, eating nutritional foods, trying to live meaningful and useful lives, deepening relationships, having fun, and exploring our creative and spiritual sides.

Adapt an open and curious attitude when exploring these areas, and don't try all of them at once. Make changes gradually. Here are some suggestions from Pate-Willig and others:

CAUTION: Specific recommendations regarding diet, nutrition, and exercise may vary and should be evaluated and discussed with your physician.

Medical and Psychological Help. Put together your medical team with care. The treatment of hepatitis C is evolving and requires knowledge of specialized tests and treatments. Many doctors don't have much experience with hepatitis C, so find a gastroenterologist or hepatologist who does. Most medical centers have doctors who specialize in liver disease (hepatologists) or can recommend appropriate community specialists.

Although credentials are important, effective therapy may also be dependent upon the doctor–patient relationship. Make sure that the two of you are a good fit. This is a very individual matter. Do you like your doctor to tell you exactly what to do, or do you prefer to have more input in decision making? Does the doctor answer your questions fully, or seem anxious to exit? Do the nurses and receptionist seem friendly and supportive?

If you need to see a mental health professional (psychologist, psychiatrist, social worker, professional counselor), get names from friends you trust and interview a few practitioners. Ask about their backgrounds and qualifications. Make sure they have experience in dealing with issues of chronic illness. They should be graduates of an accredited master's or Ph.D. program and licensed by the state as an independent practitioner or supervised by someone who is licensed.

Keep abreast of developments in hepatitis C research. The more you know, the better your decisions will be. (See the Resources section at the back of this book.) And finally, look at your own beliefs and attitudes about illness. Otherwise, you can't decide what works for you and what doesn't. We don't choose to be sick, but we can choose how we try to handle the situation.

Resource: Bridges, William. *Transitions*. Reading: Addison-Wesley, 1980.

Resource: Flach, Frederic, M.D. *Resilience: The Power to Bounce Back When the Going Gets Tough,* New York, Hatherleigh Press, 1997.

Resource: Kushner, Harold S. *When Bad Things Happen to Good People*. New York: Avon, 1981.

Resource: Travis, John W., M.D. and Regina Sara Ryan. *Wellness Workbook*. Berkeley: Ten Speed Press, 1988.

Many studies prove the importance of support systems. The results of one well-known study reported in 1989 by psychiatrist David Spiegel and colleagues showed that women with metastatic breast cancer who attended weekly group therapy sessions lived significantly longer than those who did not.[1]

Most of us benefit from a network of informal supportive relationships. Effective support always includes a sharing of emotions and feelings—a quality of reciprocity. Each person feels heard, validated, and has a sense of being able to draw upon that support, if necessary.

Formal support groups are useful because they provide a common experience for hepatitis C patients, information-sharing, a sense of not being alone, and a safe place to share feelings.

Resource: See the Resource section at the back of this book for organizations that might sponsor support groups, or call your local hospital.

Exercise and Nutrition. Physical movement not only strengthens your body, it helps your emotional state. If you can afford it, a personal trainer with experience in chronic illness is helpful. Hospitals often have cardiac or stroke rehabilitation experts who may be able to refer you to the right professional, but you don't need money to exercise. You can walk with a friend, rent a yoga or tai chi video, or try water exercise to avoid stress on painful joints. Be creative.

For information on nutrition, see Chapter 5, Taking Care of Yourself Nutritionally.

CAUTION: Consult your doctor before you begin any exercise program or make dietary changes.

Feeling Useful/Having Fun. We need a sense of meaning and purpose in our lives. We also need to have fun and play. Look for activities that create joy, hope, and a sense of living fully. Balance is the key.

> I'd always been a workaholic, but I started to question that kind of life when I learned I had hepatitis C. I didn't even like my job!
>
> I started to try some new things like meditation. Then I got into art therapy and got really excited. One day I made a sand tray containing images of my life. In it, I put a house without a roof because my nice suburban dream had blown up. I made a monster in a cage, because I felt like a monster, and a treehouse with the goddess Diana, who was the powerful part of me. I made a bridge that meant I was trying to get somewhere—paradise, a stream, lots of unconscious images.

I changed jobs. I played more. I ate healthier foods. As I look back now, I see that I'm in paradise. I crossed the bridge!

Maria

Ask yourself these questions: What is important to me? How am I acting on the important things in my life? How can I continue to have a meaningful existence within the limits of my health and energy levels?

Resource: LeShan, Lawrence. *Cancer As a Turning Point.* New York: Penguin, 1994.

Playing helps you recapture joy. "Like humor, a good joyful experience does as much for your sense of well-being as a good physical workout," says Pate-Willig. It requires flexibility and a commitment to explore options. If you can't climb mountains anymore, investigate handicapped-accessible trails or rent travel videos. Open yourself to new experiences. If you've never explored poetry, for example, now may be the time to visit your neighborhood library.

"Learn to live mindfully," says Pate-Willig. "Ask yourself: 'Do I notice the people chattering at my dinner table, and am I grateful for my family? Do I savor the vivid colors of the vegetables I'm cutting? Do I stop for a moment during the day to notice that I feel good?'"

Exploring Your Creative and Spiritual Sides. Using the mind's capacity for healing includes visualization, relaxation, guided imagery, meditation, journal writing, and creative arts. All of these are ways to help the mind create a quieter atmosphere and to improve your quality of life.

Visualization, meditation, and relaxation create a sense of relaxed alertness and counteract the stress of daily living. Visit a bookstore and look over the tapes and videos. There are more than 30 methods, so the important thing is to find what makes you feel comfortable.

Resource: Benson, Herbert and Miriam Klipper. *The Relaxation Response.* New York: Avon, 1976.

Resource: Kabat-Zinn, Jon. *Full Catastrophe Living.* New York: Dell, 1990.

Journal writing lowers stress levels and can be your best friend in the middle of the night when there's no one else to talk to. Write quickly, don't censor yourself, and find a safe place to keep your journal.

Resource: Capacchione, Lucia. *The Well-Being Journal.* North Hollywood: Newcastle, 1989.

Creative art forms (painting, drawing, music, dance, poetry) are healing because you work with symbols and images to express feelings.

Resource: Capacchione, Lucia. *The Creative Journal.* North Hollywood: Newcastle, 1989.

At first, after the diagnosis, I went a little crazy with thera-pies. I mean, I did it all—talk therapy, yoga, you name it and I did it. I ran myself ragged keeping up with all the appoint-ments.

Finally, I decided it was too messy. I wanted to play. I took a dance weekend, and there it was. When I danced, I got to the stillness inside me. For me, dance relates to life and the creative process. Staccato movements, for example, meant I was having trouble with boundaries, with saying no. It became a metaphor for all of my life, and I began to feel healing on all levels.

Then we moved, and when I was going through boxes, guess what I found? A pair of little ballet slippers! I had completely for-gotten that as a kid I had taken dance lessons—and loved them.

Sara

Guided imagery is a specific kind of relaxation and movement using the mind's own images. Most mental health professionals who deal with illness can assist you in creating an individual tape that works for you. A prerequisite is to practice relaxation so you can access guided imagery. The technique uses all five senses and works best when it's tailored to you. Not everyone sees images, for example. If that's the case with you, the therapist will use sounds or smells instead.

> *My ALT counts were high—in the 500s, so I went on interferon. It sounds a little far out, but I started to do this white light meditation. I visualized the interferon working on the hepatitis. Then my viral counts lowered to zero.*
>
> *I visualized the interferon, like white knights assisting my immune system. B.I.S., Bill's Immune System. I saw a whole army of three million knights in shining armor!*
>
> *Bill*

Even if you don't hold formal religious beliefs, you can tap into your spirituality, says Pate-Willig. "Think back to your feelings at the birth of your child, or when you suddenly came upon a bed of glorious wildflowers. Spirituality connects you with a sense of something larger than the self."

> *If I had had to face death the year I was diagnosed, I would have felt I never lived. I was terrified, and I would have been angry with lots of regrets.*
>
> *But as I got sicker, I had to go on disability. That gave me the time to explore, and I found out I could meditate, become still, and have a connection to a higher power. Now that I've had a chance to live fully, somehow I'm not as frightened of death.*
>
> *Steve*

Illness, however, can also present a theological challenge. According to Dr. House, some patients "go through a crisis of faith. People who've gone to church all their lives may suddenly feel rejected, alone and abandoned, angry with God, or feel this illness is punishment for some unknown sin. Their social network is centered on their church, so if they lose this, they lose a lot. I recommend that they talk to their clergy or to the hospital chaplain."

"Spiritual distress," says Rev. Julie Swaney, Chaplain at the University of Colorado Health Sciences Center, "occurs when a person's faith or spirit is suddenly full of holes. Everything you believe in is gone. You've lost your value system, and you feel alone. But one of the gifts of illness is the way it opens us up to life. People reassess relationships, values, their sense of time, of what's important. Spirituality has to do with how we make meaning out of our experiences. Embrace what works for you."

Resource: Benson, Herbert, M.D., with Marg Stark. *Timeless Healing, The Power and Biology of Belief.* New York: Scribner, 1996.

Resource: Frankl, Victor E. *Man's Search for Meaning.* New York: Simon & Schuster, 1984.

Resource: Kushner, Harold S. *When All You've Ever Wanted Isn't Enough.* New York: Simon & Schuster, 1986.

Finally, one last word on being good to yourself. Take small steps to wellness slowly, over time. There is no correct formula. You may move back and forth, concentrating first on one area, then another—whatever works!

There is no grief which time does not lessen and soften.

Cicero

Reference

1. David Spiegel, M.D. *Living Beyond Limits.* (New York: Random House, 1993), p. 79.

7

Taking Care of Yourself Financially

An Overview

Hey, this hepatitis C thing is tough. I get so tired, I almost fall asleep driving my truck. I've learned to pull over and take a quick nap. Just a few minutes, then I'm okay again.

I told my bosses I had hepatitis C. They nodded and said all the right things, but hey, it doesn't matter. I still have to do my job or I'm out. And if I'm out, I don't have health insurance. Then I can't afford interferon. But if I'm on interferon, I'm tired and I'm having trouble doing the work.

It's a Catch-22 situation, all right.

Tim

LIKE TIM, you may feel too sick to work, but you can't quit because you need to hold on to your health insurance. Or you're getting so many medical bills, you're worried about paying the mortgage. Any chronic illness can put a dent in your budget.

Each one of you, however, faces a different situation. This chapter presents a general overview of financial issues and supplies you with resources to help you find your own solutions.★

We'll cover:

- Cost of Treatment
    Ongoing Medical Care
    Interferon Treatment
    Transplantation
- Private Health Insurance
    Selecting Health Insurance
    Types of Private Health Insurance:
        Managed Care or Fee-for-Service
        HMOs
        PPOs
        Fee-for-Service Plans
- Government Health Insurance
    Medicare
    Medicaid
    Veterans Administration
- When You're Too Sick to Work: Applying for Disability
    Short-Term Disability Leave
- Disability Insurance
    Social Security Disability Insurance
    Supplemental Security Income (SSI)

*Note: This chapter is an overview, not an exhaustive treatment of financial options and programs. It does not provide legal advice; always contact agencies and companies for specific information and consult a lawyer for legal advice in specific cases.

Cost of Treatment

Ongoing Medical Care Costs. If you have a chronic illness, like hepatitis C, you have to consider the cost of lifelong medical care. At the very least, you need regular exams and blood tests to monitor your liver functions. For stable patients, the minimum recommendation is an annual physical examination and blood tests twice a year. You may also need a liver biopsy every three to five years. Ask your doctor what he or she recommends.

In the past year I've had a liver biopsy and a blood clotting problem that landed me in the emergency room and intensive care unit overnight. That cost big time.

I've got health insurance, so I didn't worry until I heard at my hepatitis C support group that some insurance companies put a $1 million lifetime cap on their policies. It seemed like a fortune until I started to add up just this year's medical expenses. I finally called my company and found out my cap is $2 million. What a relief!

Susie

Interferon Treatment Costs. Interferon treatment is costly. For exact prices, you may call Schering Corporation, the manufacturer of INTRON® A (Interferon alfa-2b, recombinant) at 1-800-222-7579, or Roche Laboratories, the manufacturer of Roferon®-A (Interferon alfa-2a, recombinant), customer service at 1-800-526-0625, or Amgen, the manufacturer of INFERGEN® (Interferon-consensus), customer service at 1-800-282-6436. At the time of this writing, two additional interferons were in the process of clinical trials (Wellferon®, Glaxo-Wellcome and Alferon N®, ISI Pharmaceuticals). When these products become available for use in treatment of hepatitis C, they will each have their own customer service numbers.

Interferon therapy, including blood tests and doctors' visits, costs approximately $500 per month. The standard treatment is three injections three times per week. Sometimes a physician will increase the dosage or duration of therapy, which adds to the expense. Call your health insurance provider to find out how much of the cost it will absorb.

If you need help to pay for interferon treatment, you, your doctor, or a family member may contact the pharmaceutical company's reimbursement search and financial assistance program to see if you qualify for aid.

Resource: Call Schering's Commitment to Care℠: 1-800-521-7157. The program offers help in finding coverage, cost-sharing, and the providing of drugs to indigent people. Have this information ready when you call:

1. name and address of your prescribing physician
2. diagnosis, prescribed drug therapy, and schedule
3. financial information: recent 1040 form, pay stub, Social Security number

Resource: If your doctor has prescribed Roferon®-A, and you need help to pay for treatment, your doctor may contact the ONCOLINE Reimbursement Assistance Program: 1-800-443-6676 (Virginia residents call collect 703-391-7829).

You might also consider enrolling in a study. Pharmaceutical companies often sponsor studies of promising new treatments; in many cases if you participate the sponsor covers all costs of treatment. Be sure you understand exactly what the study involves, before you sign up for it. Ask your doctor for information or call a major research center or medical school near you. (See Chapter 10, Research Trends.)

Transplantation Costs. The hospital's financial coordinator will be on your transplant team to help you figure out how you can afford the procedure. There are many costs involved: tests and consultations before the operation, the transplant operation itself, hospitalization, and follow-up care and medications.

According to Chip Webb, Coordinator, Transplant Financial Services at the University of Colorado Health Sciences Center, the cost for liver transplantation (from admission to discharge, but not including before or after care) varies widely, from $50,000 to over $1 million. The average cost is approximately $150,000. Costs vary widely around the country.

Webb meets with patients to help them find coverage for liver transplantation. Unfortunately, not everyone can meet the financial obligations to get on the recipient list. "You have to scrutinize each patient's financial and living situation to assess if they are eligible for some type of assistance. There is no formula for everybody," he says, "because people have different comfort levels of what they are willing to sacrifice for a chance at a liver transplant. For example, some people have successfully raised thousands of dollars to get on the list, and others would prefer to die than ask for money. The idea is to present options to patients and let them choose.

"Sometimes patients are in a 'Catch-22' situation. Suppose a man has been receiving Social Security benefits for one year. In another 12 months he will have Medicare that will likely pay for a liver transplant. However, he may not have that long. If he makes over $480 a month from his Social Security or has a working spouse, then it is unlikely that he would qualify for Medicaid. I see many patients who are caught in this dilemma, and I don't always have answers for them.

"Even for those patients who have Medicaid, there may still be a problem," explains Webb. "Not all state Medicaid programs will cover a liver transplant. Colorado Medicaid will cover the transplant for hepatitis C patients, but Wyoming and Montana Medicaid, for example, currently do not cover the procedure for patients over the age of 18."

Not all private insurance policies cover transplants, and both private and government health insurance have certain criteria. For example, people who have additional medical problems, such as a heart condition, a malignancy, or HIV, may find themselves excluded from coverage.

"Patients considering transplantation should check if their insurance will pay for the immunosuppressives prescriptions that they will require to prevent rejection post-transplant," says Webb. "Most insurances will cover these drugs. Even some policies that do not cover the transplant will cover the anti-rejection regimens. Since the cost of these drugs can range from $700 to $2,000 a month, it is wise to check beforehand."

In addition to these direct costs, there are many indirect expenses involved. Patients sometimes forget to allow for organ recovery costs or travel and lodging for family members, child care, and so on. Many insurance policies have caps (maximum amounts they'll spend on a patient or a procedure). Few people can pay for the entire transplant experience from a single source.

Resource: An excellent pamphlet by UNOS (United Network for Organ Sharing) discusses a combination of possible funding sources, including insurance, COBRA extended coverage, Medicare, CHAMPUS (Civilian Health and Medical Program of the Uniformed Services), charitable organizations, public fundraising campaigns, advocacy organizations, and other resources. For a copy of *Financing Transplantation, What Every Patient Needs to Know*, call toll free 1-888-TXINFO1 (1-888-894-6361).

Resource: Another booklet, written by volunteers and distributed by the Oregon Donor Program, may be helpful. For your free copy of *Finger in the Dike, Or: How to Raise $140,000 for Organ Transplant Surgery in Less Than Four Weeks*, call 1-800-452-1369, ext. 7888.

Resource: The American Liver Foundation (ALF) has established a Liver Transplant Fund that provides professional administration, at no cost, for funds raised on behalf of patients to help pay for medical care and associated transplantation expenses. For information, call 1-800-GO-LIVER or 1-888-4-HEP-ABC.

Private Health Insurance

Selecting Private Health Insurance. When you have a chronic illness like hepatitis C, you must select your health insurance carefully:

- Read your policy before signing it. Ask questions. If there is any part you don't understand, get help.
- Make sure your plan allows you to see doctors who are experts in hepatitis C: gastroenterologists, hepatologists, and transplant physicians.
- Understand the restrictions and make sure they won't affect the quality of your care. For example, does the policy cover emergency rooms, experimental treatments, drugs like interferon? What happens if you're out of town and you need medical help?
- Is there a lifetime limit or cap on treatment or drugs? A million dollars may sound high, but is it too low for a chronic condition?
- Use common sense in assessing a medical policy. When you

have hepatitis C, you have to plan ahead for extra medical care, even though you may never need it.

- Check to see if your policy pays based on "reasonable and customary" fee schedules. Policies that use fee schedules may not pay the entire bill if they feel that your doctor or hospital does not charge "reasonable" rates.
- Know any managed care provisions in your policy. Do you have any particular doctor or hospital that you are required to use? If you use a "preferred provider," will the insurance cover a larger share?

Types of Private Health Insurance: Managed Care or Fee-for-Service. Private health insurance policies fall into two categories: (1) managed care, or (2) fee for service. Managed care plans limit your choice of physician, but usually cost less. Managed care options include Health Maintenance Organizations (HMO) and Preferred Provider Organizations (PPO).

Fee-for-service policies usually provide the freedom to choose your doctor, but they often are more expensive. Look at the following factors when comparing cost of fee-for-service policies:

- monthly premiums—what the insurance costs each month
- annual deductible—how much you have to pay out of your pocket each year before the policy will pay benefits
- coinsurance—what percentage you have to pay that your insurance will not cover, usually 20 to 30 percent
- out-of-pocket maximum—the amount that you pay in coinsurance before the insurance company will begin to pay at 100 percent
- policy maximum—the maximum amount that insurance will pay over the lifetime of the policy

Whether you choose a managed care or traditional fee-for-service plan, be sure you understand how your plan works and the appeal process. If you're dissatisfied with your insurance policy, you may always review these issues with your State Commissioner of Insurance.

HMOs. Under HMO plans you have a primary care physician, a gatekeeper, who coordinates your care and decides if you should be referred to a specialist. This plan is the least costly but the most limiting in terms of freedom of choice. Because the goal is to keep costs at a minimum, your access to specialists, tests, medications, or hospital care may be restricted. It's important to do a thorough check on limitations.

PPOs. You may choose a doctor within the provider network and get 90 to 100 percent coverage of your costs or choose a doctor outside the network and receive a smaller percentage of the cost, usually 70 percent.

Fee-for-Service Plans. Usually, the choice of doctor is totally yours, but these plans are typically the most expensive. Patients with chronic hepatitis C who are exploring fee-for-service plans should choose a major medical policy that offers subspecialty physician services and adequate hospital coverage.

The insurance company usually pays 80 percent of the bill, and you pay 20 percent up to a total amount designated by your policy. Hospital and physician fees that the insurance company deems unreasonable may not be fully reimbursed.

Resource: For help in evaluating health insurance plans, ask for a copy of *Choosing Quality: Finding the Health Plan That's Right for You* and a list of accredited HMOs, from the National Committee for Quality Assurance at 1-800-839-6487.

Resource: Another useful booklet is *Checkup on Health Insurance Choices*, AHCPR #93-0018, by the Agency for Health Care Policy and Research: 1-800-358-9295.

Resource: In 1996, Congress passed the Health Insurance Portability and Accountability Act (Public Law #104-191), sponsored by Senators Edward Kennedy and Nancy Kassebaum. This act includes many significant health insurance reforms.

Some highlights of the act include: (1) "portability" provisions, (2) increased availability of coverage, and (3) expansion of COBRA continuation coverage benefits. The "portability" provisions are designed to eliminate the fear that employees will lose their health insurance if they change jobs.

You may request a copy of the act and its accompanying conference committee report from your U.S. representative or senator. Also, as with other legislation of this type, government agencies, such as the Labor Department, the Internal Revenue Service, and the Department of Health and Human Services, will issue regulations to implement the act's provisions. In addition, almost all states will have to make changes in state legislation to comply with the act. For information, call your state legislators and your state insurance department.

Resource: Some states have set up risk-sharing pools to enable people who are otherwise uninsurable to purchase health insurance. Colorado, for example, has the Colorado Uninsurable Health Insurance Plan (CUHIP). State insurance laws differ, so call your state insurance department for specific information. If you have difficulty locating your state insurance department, contact the National Association of Insurance Commissioners for the listing: 816-842-3600.

Government Health Insurance

CAUTION: Laws and regulations change over time. Double-check your facts with the agency involved. Only the agency itself can give you up-to-date, accurate material.

This chapter does not give legal advice and is not a substitute for the professional services of an attorney. Always consult a lawyer when legal issues are involved.

Medicare. At age 65, you may be eligible for medical insurance for hospital and other medical services. If you receive Social Security disability benefits for 24 consecutive months (see following section), you also may qualify for Medicare.

Medicare has two parts. Hospital insurance (Part A) covers inpatient hospital care. You already paid for this as part of your Social Security and Medicare taxes when you were working. Medical insurance (Part B) pays for doctors' services, prescriptions, and some outpatient facility and doctor visits. Part B is optional, and you'll be billed monthly for your premium.

Sign up for Medicare at your local Social Security office three months before you become 65, and you'll receive your Medicare card. Ask about enrollment periods. You may also want to purchase a Medigap policy (private insurance that fills in some of the "gaps" in Medicare's coverage).

Resources: Call the Social Security Administration at 1-800-772-1213 to request a copy of SSA Publication No. 05-10043, *Medicare*; Publication No. HCFA-10050, *Your Medicare Handbook*; and Publication No. HCFA 02179, *Medicare and Other Health Benefits*. If you have a low income and few resources, you may qualify for state aid to help pay for Medicare premiums and some other expenses; ask for HCFA Publication No. 02184, *Medicare Savings For Qualified Beneficiaries*.

Medicaid. Medicaid is a federal-state health program for people with low incomes. At present, the program is administered by state social services departments. To apply, call your county social services department.

Veterans Administration. For questions about medical benefits and disability, veterans may call the Veterans Administration Regional Office.

Resource: Dial this number and your call will be automatically directed to your regional office: 1-800-827-1000.

When You're Too Sick to Work: Applying for Disability

As hepatitis C progresses to the stage of cirrhosis, you may be less capable of functioning at home or on the job. In general, this occurs only in patients who have had the disease for many years and who have cirrhosis and signs of worsening liver function.

Our goal in this section is to provide you with a general overview of the available options for disability benefits and the process involved. For those who wish to consider applying for disability benefits, the process varies depending on your income, personal situation, and insurers or government programs.

CAUTION:

1. Laws and regulations change; unexpected circumstances arise. It's best to double-check your facts with the company, agency,

or organization involved. Medical social workers can help direct you to the appropriate agencies or programs.

2. Keep a file with copies of all your medical records. Begin right now, if you haven't already done so. Always keep your EOBs (Explanation of Benefits) from your insurance. The EOB is the document that explains what the medical provider and/or hospital is paid and contains a description of payment procedures.

3. Start a journal. Keep track of your symptoms and how they affect your daily tasks. This documentation will help you explain your symptoms to your doctor and will be important later if you ever have to file for disability.

4. This chapter does not give legal advice and is not a substitute for the professional services of an attorney. Consider consultation with a lawyer when legal issues or hearings are involved.

Resource: Call the American Bar Association at 312-988-5000 for your state's lawyer referral service number or check your phone book. Attorneys specialize in different areas, such as disability or insurance, so explain your specific problem.

If you can't afford a lawyer, contact your local Legal Aid Society or a law school that sponsors a student association offering free legal advice. Your local United Way may also direct you to possible sources of legal help.

Short-Term Disability Leave. Become familiar with your company's policies. Some companies offer paid short-term disability leave or allow you to use accumulated sick days. Companies usually require that a doctor accurately assess the nature of your symptoms and verify that you are disabled. The diagnosis of hepatitis C or treatment with interferon are not sufficient, in and of themselves, to necessarily justify disability.

I was exhausted when I started taking interferon. My sister had died recently, and I thought it was depression that had me so tired. My doctor told me I had beginning cirrhosis, and I was so sick I needed to take some time off from work.

I was incredulous. Taking time off was for operations! That was my own denial, my survival system. I was amazed that my company did approve leave—and I was paranoid. I expected surveillance cameras to sneak up on me. When I finally went back to work, it was part time, then full time. It was rough. I was achey; I had headaches. I just stayed in my cubicle and did what I had to do.

I was afraid of losing my job. I didn't know my rights. I thought if I had six absences in a row, I'd be out the door.

Joe

If you are an eligible employee and you or your family member (child, parent, spouse) becomes seriously ill from advanced hepatitis C, the Family and Medical Leave Act allows you to take up to 12 weeks of *unpaid* leave each year. Workers returning from leave must be restored to their original jobs or equivalent jobs with the same pay, benefits, and working conditions.

Resource: For more information and to find out if you are an eligible employee under the act, call the nearest office of the Wage and Hour Division, listed in most telephone directories under U.S. Government, Department of Labor, Employment Standards Administration. Ask for copies of these publications: WH Publication #1421, *Compliance Guide to the Family and Medical Leave Act*, U.S. Department of Labor, Wage and Hour Division, June 1993 (U.S. Government Printing Office: 1993—342-558/87203) and Fact Sheet No. ESA 93-24, U.S. Department of Labor Program Highlights, *The Family and Medical Leave Act of 1993* (U.S. Government Printing Office: 1993—353-844).

Resource: The 1990 Americans with Disabilities Act (ADA) prohibits job discrimination against "qualified individuals with disabilities." Employers covered under the act must make a "reasonable accommodation" for such persons depending on the particular facts in each case and on whether or not it imposes "due hardship" on the employer. "Reasonable accommodations" apply to the area of attendance and leave policies. To see if the ADA covers you and your employer and to get more specific information on the provisions of the act, call the President's Committee on Employment of People with Disabilities Information Line (Job Accommodation Network) at 1-800-232-9675 or the ADA Technical Assistance Center at 1-800-949-4232.

Resource: You can obtain ADA information, assistance, and copies of ADA documents supplied by the Equal Employment Opportunity Commission and the Department of Justice from any of the ten Regional Disability and Business Technical Assistance Centers across the country. For copies of EEOC-BK-15, *The Americans with Disabilities Act, Questions and Answers* and EEOC-BK-18, *The Americans with Disabilities Act, Your Employment Rights as an Individual With a Disability*, call 1-800-949-4232.

Disability Insurance

If you're self-employed, you may have paid for your own individual disability insurance. If you work for a company, find out if you are eligible to enroll in your company's group disability coverage. Read the terms of coverage carefully.

> *When I went on disability, I was at my highest earning capacity. It's a good thing I couldn't take a less stressful job at my company for less money. I would have had to quit anyway, and then I would have shot myself in the foot because my disability was computed as a percentage of my paycheck. It's hard enough to live on what I did get—60 percent of what I was earning.*
>
> *Arthur*

Two Social Security Administration programs offer assistance if you have to file for disability: Social Security Disability Insurance and Supplemental Security Income (SSI).

CAUTION: Brief descriptions of the programs follow, but only the agency itself can give you up-to-date, accurate material. *Call the Social Security Administration and ask them to send you infor-*

mation about disability programs: 1-800-772-1213. You can speak to a service representative between the hours of 7 a.m. and 7 p.m. on business days. Hearing-impaired callers using TTY equipment can call 1-800-325-0778 during the same hours.

Social Security Disability Insurance. This insurance covers workers (and their children or surviving spouses). In order to qualify for this disability coverage you must have worked long enough and recently enough to have made sufficient contributions to your Social Security account. Adults must have a physical and/or mental problem that prevents them from working for at least a year or that is expected to result in death. Benefits continue until a person is able to work again on a regular basis.

You may file a claim by phone, mail, or by visiting the nearest Social Security office. The claims process can take anywhere from 60 to 90 days while the agency obtains medical information and decides if the disability affects your ability to work. You'll be asked to provide your Social Security number and proof of age; names, addresses, and phone numbers of doctors, hospitals, clinics, and institutions that treated you and dates of treatment; names of all medications you are taking; medical records from your doctors, therapists, hospitals, clinics, and caseworkers; laboratory and test results; a summary of where you worked in the past 15 years and the kind of work you did; a copy of your W-2 Form (Wage and Tax Statement), or if you are self-employed, your federal tax return for the past year; dates of prior marriages if your spouse is applying.

You should also contact the doctors and treatment facilities to let them know that Social Security will be requesting medical records. The medical report forms will ask for a medical history of your condition and how it limits your activities, test results, treatment provided, information about ability to do work-related activities, and so on.

Social Security may request medical records from your physicians and hospitals to document your disability. However, your application may be processed faster if you provide this information for them up front.

After my biopsy I had to acknowledge how sick I was. I had cirrhosis. I was so fatigued that I had no life outside of work. For the time I had left, this was not the kind of life I wanted. So I became more assertive. Instead of waiting for my doctor to suggest disability, now I suggested it.

As long as I was ambulatory, I thought I wasn't disabled. But when I put my symptoms on paper, I had to accept my feelings. I wrote about my inability to concentrate, my depression, the aches and pains, the constant headaches—and I presented the list to my doctor.

He said I was disabled, outlined restrictions, gave me a prescription, and I took it to my employer. The disability plan at our company required me to sign up for Social Security Disability Insurance also.

At first, Social Security denied my claim. I went to a lawyer for help. I wish I had gone to him earlier. He told me it wasn't unusual to be denied at first. Hepatitis C symptoms of fatigue are vague, subjective. We appealed.

Social Security asked for an independent medical evaluation. I was prepared. I had kept a log of activities I could do and those I could not do. I went armed with my biopsy report. I finally saw myself as an educator of what hepatitis C was all about. I got disability.

Nadine

The Social Security Administration recommends that you don't wait to file your claim, even if you don't have all this information right away. (There is a waiting period before benefits begin, so the sooner you apply, the better.) If you need someone's help, a family member, caseworker, or other representative can contact the agency for you.

After your application is complete, the Social Security office will review it to see if you're eligible. Then they'll send your application to the Disability Determination Services (DDS) office in your state. (Consult SSA Publication No. 05-10029, which lists five questions that determine disability.)

If the claim is approved, you'll receive a notice showing the amount of your benefit and when payments start. The amount of your benefit is based on your lifetime average earnings covered by Social Security, but benefits from other sources can affect your disability check. Your case will be reviewed periodically to see if you remain disabled. After two years from the date of onset of disability, you will be eligible for Medicare benefits, regardless of your age.

If your claim is denied, a notice will explain why. You may then fill out a request for reconsideration. If the request for reconsideration is denied, your next step is to ask for a hearing. If you are denied again, you still have two more levels of appeal.

Resource: Call the Social Security Administration at 1-800-772-1213 for copies of SSA Publication No. 05-10057, *Social Security Disability Programs Can Help* and SSA Publication No. 05-10029, *Social Security Disability Benefits*.

Resource: Jehle, Faustin F. *The Complete & Easy Guide to Social Security & Medicare, 12th Edition.* Peterborough: Fraser-Vance Publishing, 1995.

Supplemental Security Income (SSI). SSI is a Social Security Administration program that makes disability payments to adults and children with little or no income or resources. To get SSI, you must be 65 or older, blind, or disabled. According to SSA Publication No. 05-11000, *Supplemental Security Income*, disabled means you have a physical or mental problem that keeps you from working and is expected to last at least a year or to result in death.

The basic SSI payment is the same all over the country, but many states add money to your check. Call the Social Security Administration to find out what your state does.

When I applied for SSI, it was as if I was fighting against my whole value system. I had dreams that I was a gunrunner in South America. It felt as though I was doing something wrong or breaking the law.

*I was barely making it before hepatitis C, and now that I'm
exhausted all the time, I can't make it at all. What else can I do?*

Sam

If you qualify for SSI, you may be able to get other aid from
your state or county, such as Medicaid (which helps pay doctor
and hospital bills), food stamps, or other social services. Call your
local social services department or public welfare office.

If you get Medicare and have low income and few resources,
you may qualify for help with some Medicare expenses under the
Qualified Medicare Beneficiary (QMB) or Specified Low-Income
Medicare Beneficiary (SLMB) programs. Only your state can decide if you qualify.

Whether your income meets SSI requirements depends on
some very specific criteria defining what's included in income and
what's included as assets outlined in SSA Publication No. 05-
11000, *Supplemental Security Income.*

Sometimes people can get both Social Security and SSI benefits. The rules that determine if you're disabled are the same for
Social Security and SSI (refer to the previous section, Social Security Disability Insurance.) You must be unable to do any kind of
work to be considered disabled under both programs.

If you think you are eligible for SSI, the Social Security Administration recommends that you file a claim right away, even if
you don't have all the information at hand. The information you
need includes your Social Security card or a record of your Social
Security number; your birth certificate or other proof of age; information about the home where you live (such as mortgage,
lease, landlord's name); information about your income and the
things you own (such as payroll slips, bank books, insurance policies, car registration, burial fund records, etc.), and names, addresses and telephone numbers of doctors, hospitals, and clinics.

Resource: Call the Social Security Administration at 1-800-
772-1213. Hearing-impaired callers using TTY equipment, call 1-
800-325-0778. Explain why you're calling and ask for helpful
information and pamphlets, including SSA Publication No. 05-

10057, *Social Security Disability Programs Can Help*; SSA Publication No. 05-11000, *Supplemental Security Income* ; SSA Publication No. 05-10100, *Food Stamps And Other Nutrition Programs*; and Publication No. HCFA 02184, *Medicare: Savings for Qualified Beneficiaries*.

Resource: Jehle, Faustin F. *The Complete & Easy Guide to Social Security & Medicare, 12th Edition.* Peterborough: Fraser-Vance. 1995.

> *Riches serve a wise man but command a fool.*
> *English proverb*

8

Treatment for Hepatitis C
The Interferon Story and Other Anti-Virals

When I was diagnosed with hepatitis C, I panicked—especially when the doctor described interferon treatment to me. I had just read this book about how toxic our environment is, so I decided to try an alternative route: macrobiotic diet, vitamin supplements, changing my dental fillings from mercury to gold—the whole nine yards.

My ALT and AST levels went down some; the PCR test went down some. I thought I had hit the cure. But the next time I got tested, the scores crept up again. It turns out that hepatitis C spikes—up and down, high and low. I was into a much healthier lifestyle—and that was good—but I still had the virus.

I finally started interferon. My test levels went down and have stayed down. As far as I'm concerned, it's the only anti-viral game in town.

Ted

MAKING TREATMENT DECISIONS can be a stressful process. You and your doctor will work together to decide on a treatment plan. But it helps to know as much as you can about your options.

In this chapter I'll cover the following topics:

- Overview
- Interferon Therapy
    What Is Interferon?
    Who Should Take Interferon?
    Interferon Treatment
    Types of Interferon
    Measuring Response
- The Patient's Experience
    Injections
    Side Effects
- Treatment Tips from Patients
- After Interferon Treatment, What Next?
    For Nonresponders
    For Responders
    Continuing Care

Overview

As a patient with chronic hepatitis C, you may experience fatigue, loss of energy, loss of concentrating ability, and a sense of inadequacy in performing your daily activities. These symptoms, feelings, and attitudes may make you emotional or susceptible to periods of depression.

I encourage you to continue to remain physically active, pursue your occupation, socialize, and maintain proper nutrition. I also recommend regular exercise and a well-balanced diet supplemented with one multivitamin per day. (See Chapters 5 and 6 for more detailed suggestions on how to take care of yourself nutritionally and emotionally.)

Remember: Alcohol and hepatitis C don't mix. Avoid excessive alcohol intake; the combination of alcohol and hepatitis C may accelerate your liver disease. I discourage the daily drinking of alcohol or taking large amounts at any time.

However, alcohol use is socially acceptable, so many patients ask me if they can take a drink once in a while. If you're not willing to abstain completely from alcohol, you should at least limit your alcohol intake to less than two ounces a week.

Patients also question me about alternative therapies. A number of herbal remedies, teas, potions, over-the-counter products, and even acupuncture claim to be effective in treating liver disease and viral hepatitis, but none have been adequately studied. The use of these treatments to eradicate hepatitis C is not encouraged because their effectiveness is doubtful and their safety, in general, is unknown. In one recently published report, a Chinese herbal remedy marketed as a sedative and analgesic, Jin Bu Huan, was associated with severe liver injury in seven patients. Be sure to check with your doctor before taking any over-the-counter products or other substances.

Interferon Therapy

What Is Interferon? Scientists identified interferon in 1957 by demonstrating that cells infected with a virus secreted a substance that had the ability to protect other uninfected cells from becoming infected. This substance, interferon, is a naturally occurring protein whose name is derived from its ability to interfere with viral replication.

Since these early studies, the interferon story has become increasingly complex. We now have three classes of interferons: alpha, beta, and gamma. Gamma interferon is ineffective against hepatitis C. Beta interferon is less effective than alpha interferon. Alpha interferons are the most effective interferons in treating patients with hepatitis C.

Who Should Take Interferon? The criteria for selecting patients for treatment were developed in the first two controlled studies of interferon in treating hepatitis C (US Multicenter Trial and NIH Trial, November 1989). These criteria center on three main issues: how long you've had the disease (chronicity), confirmation of a diagnosis of hepatitis C, and absence of severe liver injury (compensated liver disease). Therefore, patients selected for treatment should have:

- persistently elevated ALT (1.5 times normal levels) for at least six months
- liver biopsy compatible with diagnosis of chronic hepatitis
- no other serious underlying medical condition
- no evidence of hepatic failure (ascites, variceal bleed, encephalopathy)
- bilirubin < 4 milligrams/deciliter
- albumin > 3 grams/deciliter
- prothrombin time < 3 seconds prolonged beyond control
- platelet count > 70,000/microliter
- white blood count > 3,000/microliter, polymorphonuclear leucocytes (PMN) > 1,500/ microliter
- hemoglobin > 11 grams/deciliter

(For a full explanation of technical terms listed above, see Chapter 2.)

Patients should have no evidence of other underlying primary liver disease (autoimmune chronic active hepatitis or active alcoholic hepatitis, in particular). Current treatment trials and standard-of-care also require that patients test positive for the hepatitis C virus by antibody or HCV-RNA assay.

Interferon Treatment. Standard interferon therapy is prescribed as three million units (or nine micrograms for INFER-GEN®) given three times a week (usually Monday, Wednesday, and Friday) for six to 12 months. Investigators have tried higher doses and longer courses of interferon with some improvements in overall response rates. For example, pediatric patients, who receive a relatively higher dose of interferon than adults under current treatment protocols, have a higher initial response and are more likely to sustain their response in long-term follow-up.

Interferon-alfa-2b (INTRON® A, Schering-Plough) was the first interferon approved by the Food and Drug Administration (FDA) in the United States for the treatment of chronic hepatitis C. Recently, Interferon-alfa-2a (Roferon-A®, Roche) and Interferon-consensus (INFERGEN®, Amgen) have also been approved. (Table 8 lists other interferons under review either by the FDA or in clinical trials.)

TABLE 8. TYPES OF INTERFERON.
Listed in order of introduction to market.

Type	Trade Name	Pharmaceutical
Interferon-alfa-2b	INTRON® A	Schering-Plough
Interferon-alfa-2a	Roferon® A	Roche Laboratories
Interferon-consensus	INFERGEN®	Amgen
Interferon-alfa-n1	Wellferon®	Glaxo-Wellcome
Interferon-alfa-n3	Alferon-N®	Interferon Sciences, Inc.

Types of Interferon. In the next few years it is likely that the FDA will approve additional interferons and other anti-virals developed for treatment of hepatitis C. Existing data suggest that the alpha interferons are similarly effective in terms of the overall response rates of hepatitis C. Side effects are similar but their frequency of occurrence varies slightly among the different interferons.

Measuring Response. Three factors appear to consistently predict a complete or sustained response:

- The patient has an HCV genotype other than type 1 (Figure 8A).
- Plasma levels of HCV are below one million copies per milliliter.
- Liver biopsy does not show signs of cirrhosis.

FIGURE 8A. HCV GENOTYPE AND INTERFERON RESPONSE.

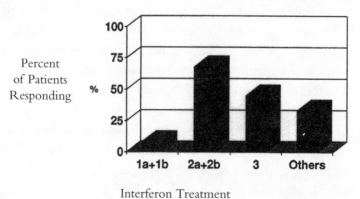

Interferon Treatment

(Some studies, but not all, suggest that young age also helps predict a positive response to interferon.)

How do you know when interferon is working? We measure its effectiveness in three ways:

1. ALT levels become normal. Hepatitis C is a liver disease, and the ALT reflects ongoing injury to the liver. Normalization of ALT implies that liver injury has stopped or is diminished. All trials commonly use ALT as a measure of effectiveness; it serves as a standard for comparing the results among trials.

The following two secondary measurements are more direct ways of assessing the anti-viral effects of treatment:

2. The hepatitis C virus (HCV-RNA) disappears from the blood, as measured by PCR assays.
3. A post-interferon treatment biopsy shows an improvement in the condition of the liver.

Unfortunately, not all experimental trials have included the last two measurements (PCR assays and liver biopsies), so we can't completely compare the results among all studies.

Looking at experimental statistics gives us important information, but when you are the person who's taking interferon, you want to know how to measure success or failure. Physicians have a special vocabulary they use to describe response:

• **Complete responder:** The patient has a normal ALT in the last two months of a course of treatment. Although there are exceptions, normalization of ALT is usually associated with the disappearance of the hepatitis C virus from the blood and an improvement in liver histology. At the end of a course of alpha interferon 30 to 60 percent of patients have a normal ALT and approximately 80 percent of those with a normal ALT will be free of virus in their blood.

- **Partial responder:** The patient experiences a partial or near-complete response to interferon. They do not normalize their ALT, but they do experience a sustained decrease in ALT of more than 50 percent of their baseline ALT (the ALT they had before treatment began). At the end of treatment, they have an ALT less than 1.5 times greater than the upper limit of normal. Most of these people fail to clear hepatitis C; when they stop interferon, their ALT usually returns to pre-treatment levels.
- **Non-responder:** Fifty percent of patients do not respond to interferon at all.
- **Sustained response/relapse:** Fifty percent of complete responders will relapse within six months after the end of treatment. The patients who do not relapse are said to have a sustained response. The length of post-treatment follow-up has varied considerably among studies, from six to 36 months. Only five to 25 percent of initially treated patients will remain ALT-normal and HCV-RNA-negative once interferon has been discontinued. One large meta-analysis suggested that both higher dose (five million units of interferon) and longer duration of treatment (12 months or more) are associated with higher rates of sustained response.
- **Disappearance of the virus (HCV-RNA):** Patients who

FIGURE 8B. ALT AND HCV–RNA PROFILE OF
A COMPLETE RESPONDER

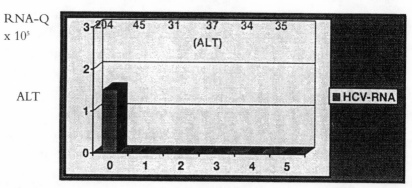

Months on Interferon

achieve a normal ALT may also find that their levels of hepatitis C virus go down to zero (see Figure 8B). It is possible that patients who continue to have a normal ALT and negative HCV-RNA may be cured of hepatitis C.

- **Improved liver histology:** In most studies, interferon therapy is associated with improvement in the condition of the liver cells. Improved histology is due mostly to reduced inflammatory activity. Recent studies also suggest that interferon therapy may inhibit the production of substances that cause liver fibrosis.

The Patient's Experience

Most patients are nervous about interferon injections and concerned about dealing with side effects of treatment.

Injections. In my experience, patients quickly learn how to give themselves injections. Most people think of the deep muscle injections they get for flu shots, and they panic about doing this to themselves. Interferon injections are much easier to administer because they are subcutaneous. Subcutaneous means you have to get the needle only under the skin and not deep into muscle.

> *I was really nervous about learning how to give myself a shot. When I came into the office, the nurse was looking all around for an orange to practice on. She never did find it. So we used the pad on the exam table, then a tissue box. It was funny, and it made me laugh—something I never expected to happen.*
>
> *The first couple of times I did it myself at home, I put the needle in too horizontally. I was going push, push, push and nothing happened. I got awful bruises.*
>
> *Back to the nurse. She told me to pinch my skin between two fingers, hold the syringe like a dart and go in straight at a 90° angle. That worked!*
>
> Marla

It's important that you ask questions and practice injections under a nurse's supervision until you feel comfortable. You should be taught about refrigerating and mixing the drug, sterile technique, how to pick injection sites, and how to dispose of needles. Be sure to ask for the helpful teaching material and videotapes that pharmaceutical companies give to physicians for their patients' use.

I recommend that the first shot be given in the office. Although it's highly unlikely for a patient to have an immediate adverse reaction, we observe the patient for a couple of hours.

Side Effects. Each person reacts differently to interferon. The most common complaints are flu-like symptoms. Why? When you get an actual case of the flu, your body fights back by sending interferon to attack the invader. Interferon is at least partially responsible for the tired, achy, and feverish symptoms.

Some people don't have many symptoms during interferon treatment; other people get chills, muscle aches, nausea, even diarrhea. These symptoms usually subside after the first few weeks. Weight loss is also a common side effect, but it tends to persist throughout the course of therapy. Some patients are able to maintain their weight and improve their energy by using supplements, such as Ensure Plus®, Resource®, and Suplena®.

To help with side effects, I recommend two regular strength Tylenol® just before you take the injection. Side effects may also be reduced if you're well hydrated before and after the injection (two glasses before an injection and about two-and-a-half quarts of fluid a day).

For fatigue, it may help to have a daily nap or rest period. Paradoxically, some patients feel their fatigue is relieved by daily activity, including exercise. Eat small, more frequent meals if you're losing your appetite. To avoid skin reactions, rotate the injection sites.

During interferon therapy you will need frequent blood tests. The main reason for doing these blood tests is to be certain your blood counts are adequate. Interferon reduces the white blood cell count and the platelet count. This effect of interferon is directly related to the dose used; higher doses cause a greater lowering of the counts. Sometimes the dose of interferon may need to be reduced or even discontinued.

Particularly distressing side effects that occur in a minority of patients include depression, mental changes, and hair loss. Depression on interferon usually occurs in patients with a pre-treatment history of depression. However, it can occur in any patient, bears close supervision, and may require reducing the dosage or even stopping treatment. In some cases, in order to continue interferon, your physician may prescribe medication to control symptoms of depression (Zoloft®, Elavil®, Effexor®, or Prozac®). If hair is lost during treatment, it usually grows back after treatment stops. Your physician will monitor you closely to watch out for other rare side effects, including thyroid disease or the development of other autoimmune disorders (see Chapter 4).

Be sure to tell your doctor if any of these symptoms appear:

- thoughts of suicide
- thoughts of homicide
- sustained fever (greater than 102° F) or other signs of infection
- generalized rash
- any symptoms that are interfering with your daily activity

Interferon may affect your ability to fight infection. Do not undergo procedures, such as excessive dental work, without checking with your doctor first; your physician may decide to prescribe an antibiotic to protect you.

Generally, most people adjust well. I tell patients to keep busy, exercise, drink lots of water, rest when they need to, socialize. Focus on positive things. Above all, don't let interferon isolate you.

Treatment Tips from Patients

Here are some tips from hepatitis C patients who've gone through the interferon process. Remember, what works for one person may not work for you. Once you become familiar with this drug, you'll find your own comfort level.

For me, drinking lots of water helped. If I didn't stay hydrated, I felt worse.

Elane

When my husband started interferon, it changed our lives. We weren't prepared for it. Interferon can be hard on the spouse, too. To be supportive, I had to plan things at a slower rate.

My husband and I used to ski all day long—black and double-black runs. We used to take 10 to 15 mile hikes. During treatment, I would have to encourage him to take a half-hour walk on flat ground—just to get him off the couch and outside.

Martha

I dropped 20 pounds because I had no appetite—and I'm pretty thin as it is. My stomach was ... I don't know, I just couldn't seem to eat. You really have to make sure you eat, even if you have to take several smaller meals throughout the day.

Now that I'm off interferon, I'm drinking two of those instant breakfast mixes each day, and I've gained back 12 pounds!

Elliot

I'm on five million units, and I'm able to continue to ride my bike 200 miles a week. If I can't ride, the effects of the interferon seem stronger.

Nat

The people in my support group decided the two major things that helped were to get a lot of rest and to have a positive attitude. What's really interesting is that in spite of the side effects, no one was sorry they had tried interferon.

Cassie

Here's a tip that works for me. Take your thumb and press hard for 10 seconds on the place where you're going to inject. It numbs the skin a little bit.

Della

They told me to take the interferon at bedtime, so I'd sleep through the worst part. But that didn't work well for me; I kept waking up. Now I take it at about 6 or 7 p.m., and I get a good night's rest.

                                                                    Stu

I'm a fair bit more irritable. So I apologize and say I'm not feeling well. It's me, not you. I do a fair amount of apologizing.

                                                                    Dick

I had a terrible time at first—and I'm not a wimp. I'm very athletic; exercise is a big part of my life. But my hands swelled up. I had awful joint pains—so bad that I had to give up golf. I couldn't hold the club!

Then my enzyme counts went down, and I knew I was a responder. The medication for the swelling started to work, too. Now that I know the interferon is helping, my attitude's changed. I look forward to each shot. I want those counts to keep going down—and I'm golfing again.

                                                                    Lewis

The biggest thing that bothers me is fatigue, low energy. I used to go back-country skiing, but now it's so much work that I have to stop frequently. Also, I get headaches. I never was a person who got them before.

                                                                    Gay

It's a peculiar kind of headache. I call it the interferon headache. Also, it seems as though I'm more forgetful. All my friends tell me they forget things, too, that I'm just getting older. But it seems different to me. Now I write everything—and I mean everything—down!

                                                                    Alma

I never had the symptoms that other people report, except for feeling more tired than usual. I felt okay. Still, it was great getting off the interferon. I noticed the difference.

                                                                    George

One night I took an early bath and really soaked. Then I did the shot. My skin was so soft, the needle went right in. Don't do the reverse, though. Don't take a hot bath after the shot.

Hallie

In the morning and at night, I feel nauseous. If I eat, the nausea goes away. I have to concentrate on eating. And if I eat right before or after an injection, I don't have side effects.

Mandy

My hairdresser told me my hair was thinning out, but not to worry because it was so thick in the first place. When I stopped interferon, it all came back.

Bernie

For me, the fatigue is the tough part. I got over the slight fever and upset stomach in the first couple of days. But I do get tired, and I just have to rest more. About midway through the treatment, I had to go on an antidepressant, and that's helped me a lot.

Jay

I've had to learn to say no. It's amazing how you can simplify your work life if you have no choice. And I've learned not to schedule too many appointments in one day. If I'm running from one thing to another, I'm wiped out at the end of the day.

Kari

After Treatment, What Next?

When you finish the course of interferon your doctor prescribes, you'll know if you're a nonresponder or a responder. Nonresponders, including partial responders, fail to sustain a normal ALT in the last two months of interferon therapy, while the complete responder maintains the normal ALT on treatment. What your doctor recommends next depends on your initial response to treatment.

If You Are a Nonresponder. For nonresponders, the first question is whether you took the interferon as prescribed. Did you miss doses? If so, why? Were the side effects intolerable? Were you able to take the full dose or was the dosage reduced? If the dosage was reduced, why? The answers to these questions tell the physician how to proceed.

If you missed doses and never received a full course of treatment, the simplest recommendation may be to consider a full standard course of interferon. Some patients, however, experience intolerable side effects, and they can't comply with treatment. When that's the case, simply retreating at the same dose isn't a likely option unless other treatment can minimize side effects. For example, if the dosage was reduced or stopped due to depression, it may be possible to retreat with interferon after treating the depression. If the dose was reduced because of severe lowering of white blood cells or platelets, you will probably not tolerate retreatment with interferon.

Doctors must address these and other issues because current protocols involving retreatment with interferon usually use higher doses and for longer duration, or the combination of interferon plus ribavirin. Obviously, patients intolerant to interferon therapy are not likely to tolerate these retreatment protocols.

Should you consider a higher dose, longer duration retreatment? Standard interferon therapy is three million units three times a week for six months. Investigators have tried several other doses and durations. If one analyzes a large number of these trials (more than 3,000 treated patients), the results suggest that doses of five million units or more or durations of 12 months or more are associated with higher rates of complete and sustained response. In contrast, a recent U.S. trial examining a wide range of doses of interferon administered for either six or 12 months failed to demonstrate a convincing advantage of either higher dose or longer duration. Nonetheless, most investigators currently recommend these changes to treatment protocols.

Other options for retreatment include new interferons. We now have only three FDA-approved interferons to treat hepatitis

C: INTRON® A (Schering), Roferon®-A (Roche), and INFERGEN® (Amgen). Soon, the FDA may approve several new ones for treating chronic hepatitis C: Wellferon® (Glaxo-Wellcome) and Alferon® (ISI). Perhaps some patients who failed to respond to interferon-alfa-2b will respond to treatment with one of the other interferons.

Results from small trials have suggested that ribavirin, a nucleoside analogue with antiviral activity against RNA viruses, may enhance the response to interferon even though it is ineffective against hepatitis C when given alone. Adding ribavirin to interferon may double the long-term sustained response rate in patients who are taking interferon for the first time and in patients who responded initially to interferon but then relapsed. Some nonresponders to interferon mono-therapy may experience a complete response when treated with this combination, but the overall outcome for nonresponders is not yet known and is currently under investigation.

If You Are a Responder. For responders, a sustained response is the most desirable outcome after interferon treatment. That is, you experience a complete response on treatment (normal ALT), and you sustain the complete response even after interferon is withdrawn. Most patients with a sustained response have also cleared the virus from their blood and have improvement in their liver biopsy (fewer inflammatory cells and less damage).

Long-term sustained responders (more than three years) may have halted the progression of their liver disease and may have actually cleared hepatitis C completely. However, there is always the risk that hepatitis C may only be dormant and reactivate, flaring at a later date. Patients should continue to undergo periodic biochemical tests and physical examinations.

Unfortunately, the majority of patients with a complete response will relapse when followed for six to 12 months after treatment. Relapse does not usually show itself in symptoms; it's detected by an increase in ALT. Patients who relapse typically respond to retreatment with interferon. We don't yet know whether these patients are best treated by higher doses, longer duration, or the combination of interferon with ribavirin.

Continuing Care. Patients with hepatitis C are at risk for progressive liver injury, cirrhosis, complications of end-stage disease, and may ultimately require liver transplantation for survival. Additionally, these patients are at risk for developing liver cancer (hepatoma). Thus, general medical advice includes ongoing physical examinations by a physician and biochemical tests of liver function. Cirrhotic patients with hepatitis C may need periodic measurement of alpha-fetoprotein and ultrasound examinations to detect early liver cancer. You should understand that the combination of alcohol and hepatitis C can cause early progression to cirrhosis and liver failure. Active alcoholism is a contraindication to liver transplantation.

> *A drug is a substance which when injected*
> *into a guinea pig produces a scientific paper.*
>
> *Anonymous*

9

Liver Transplants
A Miracle of Modern Medicine

I was on the liver transplant waiting list for—oh, gosh—nine months. Finally, they gave me a pager because it was getting close. The second day, early in the morning, I was sleeping in that ozone where you're just starting to wake up, when I heard the pager go off. I bolted out of bed. I hadn't moved like that for months because I'd been so sick.

I reached for my pager, but it wasn't blinking. My heart was just pounding! Then I heard the garbage truck in the alley; it was the warning beep as the truck backed up.

The real call came three weeks later at 4:30 a.m. The doctors kept asking me if I was afraid, if I was sure I wanted to do this. "My God, yes!" I said. "Let's get this show on the road."

Tom

SOME PEOPLE with hepatitis C develop cirrhosis, liver failure, and need a liver transplant to survive. Liver transplantation is the most complicated therapy for people with end-stage hepatitis C, but it produces seemingly miraculous results.

Pre-transplant patients go through a difficult time. They suffer from a variety of symptoms, including jaundice, sleeplessness, itching, fluid buildup, mental confusion, and hemorrhaging. A successful transplant cures these symptoms, and the patient goes on to lead a full, productive life.

This chapter covers the following topics:

- Liver Transplantation: A Brief History
- When Do You Need a Liver Transplant?
  The Most Common Diagnosis: Hepatitis C
  Signs That You Need a Transplant
  Denial of Transplants
  Paying for Transplants
- The Transplant Team
- Waiting for a Liver
  The Evaluation Process
  Transplant Support Groups
- Liver Transplant Surgery
  Donor Livers
  Living-Related Liver Transplant
  The Surgical Procedure
  The Hospital Stay
- Living with a New Liver
  Medications to Prevent Rejection
  Managing Complications
  Psychological Transformation
- Improved Survival Rates
- How Organs Are Allocated
  UNOS
  Centers of Excellence

Liver Transplantation: A Brief History

The first liver transplant was performed by Dr. Thomas Starzl in 1963 at the University of Colorado in Denver. In 1983, a National Institutes of Health (NIH) consensus conference on the therapeutic role of liver transplantation concluded, "After extensive review and consideration . . . liver transplantation is a therapeutic modality for end-stage liver disease that deserves broader application."

At that time, only six centers in North America and four in Europe performed hepatic transplantation. Ten years later, 3,442 patients had the procedure at 88 centers in the United States. As of February 19, 1997, there were 7,684 patients on the active U.S. waiting list.

Who Gets a Liver Transplant?

The Most Common Diagnosis: Hepatitis C. Liver transplantation is the most successful therapy for patients with a wide array of diseases that ultimately result in liver failure. The most common diagnosis for transplant is cirrhosis due to chronic hepatitis C. Laennec's cirrhosis, caused by alcohol, ranks second, but co-infection with hepatitis C is common in these patients— illustrating once again that the combination of alcohol and hepatitis C speeds the progression of liver disease.

Signs That You Need a Transplant. Obvious clinical signs and symptoms usually accompany advanced liver disease, including:

- ascites (accumulation of fluid in the abdomen)
- encephalopathy (alteration of mental function)
- variceal hemorrhage (bleeding from veins in the esophagus or stomach)
- worsening nutritional status
- diminishing quality of life

Patients who have a spontaneous infection in the ascites fluid, low serum albumin (< 2.8 grams/deciliter), clotting problems (prothrombin time > 5 seconds prolonged), and severe sustained jaundice should be given urgent consideration for transplantation. All of the above findings indicate severe liver dysfunction and are late signs of end-stage liver disease.

I found out I had hepatitis C when I came to the hospital a year ago. I had a lot of fluid in my stomach. They drained me and sent me home. I couldn't sleep. I'd lay down, stand up. The only way I could get some sleep was to fill the bathtub up so I could get some buoyancy, which relieved the pain in my stomach.

The second time I had to go to the hospital, they did an ultrasound. That's how I found out I needed a transplant.

Chris

Many people with cirrhosis have few or no findings of liver disease. Doctors say that these patients have "compensated" cirrhosis, and that it may be too early to consider liver transplantation. However, the waiting list for liver transplants is expanding, while the pool of donors is staying about the same. Patients often wait on the list for one, two, or more years before they get a liver.

Once you have cirrhosis, your doctor must monitor your blood tests closely and watch for any physical signs of decompensation in order to time the referral for liver transplantation. Unfortunately, not all patients with compensated cirrhosis are the same; some will remain stable for several years, but others may deteriorate relatively rapidly.

The course of hepatitis C varies greatly, so your physician must make an imperfect estimate of your chances of having a life-threatening complication over a one- to two-year follow-up period. If your doctor estimates that you have more than a 20 percent chance of sustaining such a complication, you should be evaluated for transplantation.

Denial of Transplants. You will be denied a liver transplant if you have AIDS, incurable cancer, active infection in the blood, active alcohol abuse, or severe underlying heart, lung, or multi-organ disease. If you have had prior extensive abdominal surgery, a clotted portal vein, extensive liver cancer, an isolated liver cancer larger than five centimeters, cancer of the bile ducts, or active hepatitis B, you might be excluded from transplantation.

Paying for Transplants. See Chapter 7, Taking Care of Yourself Financially.

The Transplant Team

Liver transplantation is a complex procedure requiring many specialists to care for you. Usually, your transplant team consists of a hepatologist, a hepatology nurse, a transplant surgeon, a transplant anesthesiologist, a transplant nurse coordinator (who keeps you informed and tells you when a liver becomes available), a social worker (who provides you and your family with emotional support), a psychiatrist (who meets with you and your family to evaluate your strengths and weaknesses and make recommendations to help you through the transplant experience), a nutritionist (who deals with pre-transplant issues, such as overweight problems or nutritional wasting, and helps with recommendations for your post-transplant nutritional needs), and a financial coordinator.

Waiting for a Liver

The Evaluation Process. You will be asked to take many diagnostic tests and meet with a psychiatrist and social worker. Usually, you meet with each person on the transplant team. The process can take a couple of days. When all the tests and interviews are completed, the team meets to approve or deny your candidacy for transplantation and may suggest additional evaluations or consultations.

> *I had two days of evaluation, from early morning until 5 o'clock in the evening. The tests were tough, but I got a lot of kindness and attention. I met everybody—the psychiatrist, the surgical team. I had to bring my whole family to the social worker. Oh boy, I've never had such tests. At my first stop, they took 21 vials of blood!*
>
> *They were very frank with me. They wouldn't waste a liver if other things were wrong with me. My previous doctor had told me I was too old to get a liver. I'm 61. The transplant team said I checked out to be in pretty good health for my age, and now I'm on the waiting list.*
>
> *Carla*

At my evaluation, the psychiatrist must have asked me ten times if I was a closet drinker. I know they have to find out if you're an active alcoholic, but I found it offensive. Everyone assumes that you're an alcoholic if you need a liver transplant. That's the first thing you have to overcome.

Bea

When they asked me why I thought I should get a transplant, I said, "I have seven grandchildren. I have much to teach and share. When I get my liver, as soon as I'm able, I intend to educate people and speak to people about becoming donors."

Leonora

In trying to evaluate your ability to tolerate transplant surgery, the transplant team will give you some diagnostic tests. Depending on your condition, the tests may include blood tests, colonoscopy (view of the entire colon through a colonoscope), CT scan (a radiologic test that lets doctors see the anatomy and size of your liver), ECG (an electrocardiogram), endoscopy (a procedure that allows doctors to look for ulcers or bleeding in the esophagus or stomach), ERCP (a procedure performed when there is concern about blockage or narrowing in the bile ducts), flexible sigmoidoscopy (a procedure that lets the physician look at the lower colon for polyps, hemorrhoids, ulcers, and colon or rectal cancer), pulmonary function tests (a breathing test that measures the function of your lungs), and ultrasound (a test that gives information about the size and shape of your liver through sound waves). If you have conditions that require additional tests, you may be asked to meet with a consultant, such as a cardiologist.

The Waiting List. Once you're placed on the list, you can wait from a few months to more than two years for a donor liver. This is an incredibly difficult period of waiting apprehensively while having to deal with life changes, physical symptoms, and financial changes. If you're the major breadwinner who can't go to work, you may lose the social network from your job.

Life is on hold. I haven't had too many problems, except mentally—I worry a lot. The toxins make your mind goofy. I can't remember things or make good judgments.

And it's hard on my wife. This mental problem has been developing over years, and we didn't know why, so we've had a lot of marital problems. We go to counseling, and we've learned to fight fair, but she's scared of the hepatitis C. She doesn't have any desire to be intimate with me at all. It's pretty hard.

It's hard for me to accept knowing that I'm dying. I only have 10 to 15 percent usage of my liver. I've been in and out of the hospital five times. Sometimes I wonder if I'll die before I get a liver.

Thomas

I've been on the waiting list for seven months. It's like an out-of-body experience—as if it's happening to someone else, not to me. Sometimes I realize I have lots to get in order, because a percentage of people don't make it. You want a liver to come, and yet you don't.

Normally, I can battle the depression, but last night I couldn't sleep. I tossed and turned. When that happens, I start cooking. I love to cook.

Johanna

I waited 515 days for my liver—and each day was a little more painful and difficult than the day before.

I think the secret of my success during surgery was maintaining a positive attitude. I packed my suitcase in August with a red flannel robe and a Santa Claus hat. It was hot, and I felt lousy, so why did I pack for Christmas?

I was baking Christmas cookies with my grandchildren when the phone rang. Laughing and covered from head to toe in flour, I asked my husband to tell whoever it was that I was too busy for a transplant. It was the call from the hospital. I got my liver that night.

Deanne

It's critical at this stage to talk about your struggles with a good friend or therapist. Keeping a personal journal is helpful. You are going through a fundamental shift in how you think of yourself and preparing for the psychological changes of the transplant.

Transplant Support Groups. Transplant support groups can be a source of strength and encouragement for pre- and post-transplant patients. The long waiting period, difficult symptoms, the trauma of surgery, the psychological shift of accepting another person's organ—all of these issues are unique to transplant patients. No one else can truly understand what it's like.

I feel a lot more comfortable in the support group now than I did six months ago. Getting to know the people, being involved with their lives, and caring for each other have helped.

When people get their transplants, it's like day and night. I look at myself as night, and they're day. Sam, he just got his. I watched him go through his struggle, and he looked really bad. It's amazing what a new liver can do for a person. It's a shot in the arm. Their facial expressions change. They glow.

Chris

I feel happier, less depressed. I don't participate a lot in the group, but I'm learning. When I get my transplant, I'll go to the group because it seems to be a help to new people who come in.

Juan

The tiredness, not sleeping, itching—no one else can know how bad you feel. They wouldn't believe it if you told them. You need to talk, to vent. If I talked to my family, I'd cry and they'd cry. You don't need that. How you feel is how you feel.

Shelley

It helped me to see others waiting. I was a basket case, but I began to accept that it was going to happen. I'd get my liver.

Pete

I cried at the group the first time I went. To see all those people—it was overwhelming. For the first time, my husband felt positive about the transplant. He had been reluctant to have me go through it, but he saw so many people looking so good and doing so well.

Alicia

I think everyone should be required to go to a transplant support group. At first I dug my heels in and refused to go. I had the feeling I was assisting Mother Nature and wondered whether I had the right to do that. When I saw others in the support group, I decided if I could have that quality of life back, I'd go for it.

Terry

Your transplant team can refer you to a support group, or you can check the resources listed at the end of this chapter. In addition to support groups, many people tell me they find it helpful to read about other liver transplant patients' experiences and about the procedure itself. Here are some books my patients recommend:

Resource: Maier, Frank with Ginny Maier. *Sweet Reprieve.* New York: Crown, 1991.

Resource: McCartney, Scott. *Defying the Gods.* New York: Macmillan, 1994.

Resource: Starzl, Thomas E. *The Puzzle People.* Pittsburgh: University of Pittsburgh, 1992.

Liver Transplant Surgery

Donor Livers. In most states, you can sign an organ donor permission statement on your driver's license; a witnessed signature is a legal form of consent. Most organ procurement organizations, however, request additional consent from the closest living relative. These organizations identify potential donors by interacting with emergency rooms and intensive care units.

Organ donation is one of the highest forms of giving and caring, and the vast majority of religious denominations endorse it.

The generosity of organ donation makes possible the miracle of transplantation. Here is Judy Ferrin's story:

> At the hospital, the doctors diagnosed my daughter, Allison, with toxic shock syndrome. She went from laughing and joking with me to sleeping, a coma, and dying within 24 hours. She was 19 years old.
>
> Just three weeks before, the two of us were watching a little boy on TV who needed a new heart. We decided to donate our organs if something happened to us—so I knew what her wishes were, and I told her nurse.
>
> The night before the funeral, I tossed and turned. I felt a need to speak at the service, but I was so afraid. We got a call from the doctor that morning. They had successfully transplanted her kidneys. Other organs were also transplanted, but that was the first, the turning point. A wave of relief went over me. And I was able to speak about Allison to the hundreds of people who came to mourn with our family.
>
> When we give to other people, it helps us through our grief. It helps us as much as the people we give to.

Did you know that the liver donor usually donates as many as seven vascular organs for seven different patients? Suitable liver donors are patients under age 65 who are brain-dead but whose hearts are beating. (In some cases, donors as old as 80 have been used.) They have no underlying malignancy, and they test negative for AIDS and active hepatitis B. The donors must have stable heart function with acceptable liver tests, serum sodium less than 170, and preferably been hospitalized for fewer than seven days. Donors and recipients must match by blood type and approximate body size but not by gender. It's customary to biopsy the donor liver to be certain that it is not scarred, fatty, or severely damaged. Once recovered, the donated organs are flushed with a special solution that preserves them for up to 48 hours.

Patients frequently ask whether organs from donors who test positive for hepatitis C can be used for transplantation. Yes, but the recipient will acquire hepatitis C. One study followed 29 recipients of organs from 13 donors who tested positive for hepatitis C. Twenty-eight of the 29 recipients tested positive for hepatitis C after the transplant. For this reason, we restrict the use of these donor livers to a recipient who already has hepatitis C or to a critically ill patient in urgent need of a transplant—one placed on the United Network for Organ Sharing (UNOS) as status 1. (For more information on UNOS, see Resources at the end of this chapter.)

Living-Related Liver Transplant. You may be thinking, "By the time I need a transplant, there will be too many people on the waiting list, and I won't ever get one!" One solution for the shortage of donors may be living-related liver transplantation, where a portion of the donor's liver is removed and then transplanted. The Japanese, for example, still debate the concept of brain death, so most liver donations in Japan are from live donors. Although the majority of these transplant operations have been performed on pediatric patients, the technique has also been used in adults. It is my opinion that living-related donation will soon become commonplace in the United States.

The living donor undergoes careful medical, psychological, and social evaluation. More than one-third of potential donors are rejected because their livers are unsuitable or they have underlying medical conditions that increase the risk of complications from surgery. The risks to the donor from the liver resection (surgery) are few. Death is rare, but problems have occurred, including pulmonary emboli, gastrointestinal bleeding, bile duct injury, and infection. The portion of the liver that is removed regenerates over the next few months.

Overall outcome for recipients primarily relates to their pretransplant clinical condition. When the procedure is performed in stable patients under non-urgent conditions, the one-year survival rate is greater than 90 percent. Survival rates decrease when the transplant takes place in more urgent circumstances. Nevertheless, living-related liver transplantation may become commonplace in the future.

The Surgical Procedure. The human body has two kidneys, two lungs—but only one liver. Scientists have created artificial kidneys (kidney dialysis) and even artificial hearts, but no one has been able to duplicate the hundreds of functions of the liver to create an effective liver dialysis machine. Liver transplant surgery, therefore, has no fallback position, no margin for error.

Although the original method pioneered by Dr. Starzl has been modified, the basic technique remains essentially unchanged. The operation has three phases:

1. dissection to access the patient's liver
2. removal of the patient's liver
3. connecting the donated liver

First, the surgeon meticulously dissects tissues and promptly controls bleeding vessels to expose the patient's liver. This process takes about one to two hours. Blood loss ranges from zero to five pints of red blood cells.

In the next phase, the surgeon clamps the blood vessels supplying your liver and removes the liver. Then the surgeon and anesthesiologist work together to maintain adequate blood clotting factors. The anesthesiologist carefully monitors your blood and blood pressure to give you the proper fluids and blood products. In the last phase, the surgeon positions the donor liver in your abdomen and sews the blood vessels together. This procedure takes from one-and-a-half to three hours; blood loss ranges from zero to five pints.

Once all the vessels are connected, the surgeon must unclamp the main vessels. After unclamping, one of the more critical periods of the procedure begins—especially if your blood clotting is poor. After you stabilize, your surgeon connects your bile duct to the donor bile duct and removes the donor gallbladder.

Livers typically begin to function immediately after their blood supply is established. Clotting improves, and the liver makes bile on the operating table!

"The most critical moment in the operation," says University of Colorado's Chief of Transplantation, Dr. Igal Kam, "is when we release the clamps holding the vessels going to the new liver, and the new liver changes in color from pale or dark brown to a more pink-brown, because new blood is flowing to the liver. When we see the yellow-brown bile start to appear from the bile duct, we can relax because we know the liver is going to work. There's no room for mistakes in this procedure.

"About 40 to 50 percent of patients go off the respirator in the operating room and we can talk to them. After six to eight hours of surgery, it's great to talk to the patient. We deal with very sick people who sometimes have only hours to live. After the transplant, then we see the miracle."

The Hospital Stay. After the operation you'll be monitored in an intensive care unit (ICU) where the staff is specifically trained to manage this early post-transplant period. If you don't have any complications, you'll spend 24 to 48 hours in the ICU and then transfer to the inpatient transplant unit.

> *In intensive care I was in la-la land from the prednisone IV. For two days I thought I was in an alien spaceship. Other patients were in the ship, and that's how they were making us well. My vision was foggy. Everything sounded as if it came from a long metal tube, echoing, distorted. But I was happy, fine with that.*
>
> *When I went to a regular room, I was still foggy and doped up. It was uncomfortable, not painful. I was cranky, though—had some major mood swings. After four days, they got me moving again. On my first walk, the IV stand got away from me, and I almost fell on my face. Then I progressed to day passes—went out for a few hours and came back. I was there two-and-a-half weeks.*
>
> *Harry*

> *My legs were like tree trunks, they were so swollen with fluid. You couldn't tell I had five toes; it looked like one big toe. A week*

after the surgery, I had lost 60 pounds. The doctors would come in and tickle my toes, just for fun.

Janet

Usually, patients stay in the hospital from five to 20 days depending on their condition. Some people require extensive rehabilitation, such as physical therapy or nursing, due to their weakened situation before the transplant.

After discharge the patient is monitored in transplant outpatient clinics for a few weeks to a few months and then returns to the care of referring primary care physicians or gastroenterologists. The transplant center continues to guide patient management through close cooperation with referring physicians.

Living with a New Liver

Although highly variable from patient to patient, most people require from three to six months to physically recover from surgery and adjust to new medications. Liver transplantation is a profound event that affects every part of a patient's life—the mind as well as the body. Patients must learn to live with lifelong medications, deal with the fear of rejection of the organ, and come to terms with a profound physical and psychological transformation.

Medications to Prevent Rejection. After the transplant, you need to take medications to prevent your immune system from rejecting your new liver. The medications are called immunosuppressants and include the following: cyclosporine (Sandimmune®, Neoral®), FK506 (Prograf®), azathioprine (Imuran®), steroids (Prednisone®, Solumedrol®), mycophenolate mofetil (Cellcept®), and OKT3.

Most patients take either cyclosporine or FK506 as primary therapy, and use the other agents to strengthen the anti-rejection effect. In the first six to 12 months it's common to take two or three anti-rejection medications. After that period most patients remain on cyclosporine or FK506, either alone or in combination with low-dose Prednisone®.

*So many pills! I had eight of one kind. Taking my medica-
tion was like eating a snack. When I went to the pharmacy to pick
up my first prescription, they gave it to me in a shopping bag—
and then another little bag.*

*The bill was $1,668 the first month. Ten months later, it's
down to about $300.*

Al

Although the medications have side effects, most of them are
dose-related and respond to either lowering the dose of the specific immunosuppressant or changing to another medication.

Never change doses by yourself. All dose adjustments of immunosuppressants require the supervision of your doctor. If you
take too little immunosuppression, you run the risk of rejecting
your liver transplant. If you take too much immunosuppression,
you risk developing a serious infection.

Managing Complications. It's essential that your transplant
team supervise you closely during your post-transplant outpatient
care. Two problems patients frequently encounter are rejection
and recurrence of hepatitis C.

If rejection occurs, it typically does so within the first three
months of the transplant and is detected by a rise in liver enzymes.
Elevations of liver enzymes and bilirubin occur, although the first
change noted is usually an increase in AST. In some cases, rejection is very mild and does not require additional immunosuppressive treatment. In more severe cases of rejection, the patient may
experience fever (up to 102°F), poor appetite, fatigue, and malaise.

*When my wife had a transplant, I was more scared than she
was. I still have fear. If she gets sick, even a common cold or the flu,
I still get scared. This is our second chance; there has to be a reason.*

Roger

Nearly all rejections occur within three months of transplantation, but occasionally rejection happens later. "Late rejection"
usually results from low levels of immunosuppressive therapy due

to improper dosing, addition of a new medication, or development of a simultaneous illness such as diarrhea or liver dysfunction. Rejection usually responds to intravenous steroids or other strategies (OKT3).

Recurrent episodes of hepatitis C in post-transplant cases are often mistaken for late rejection. Recurrent hepatitis C must be carefully considered before one embarks on a course to treat rejection.

You should expect hepatitis C to infect the liver transplant. We don't yet know how to prevent this. Pre-transplant treatment with interferon often is not practical because pre-transplant patients have low white blood cell counts, low platelets, and a liver that's in poor condition. In addition, no immunoglobulin preparations exist that inactivate hepatitis C. In contrast to these negative results, one recent trial has suggested that ribavirin used with interferon after the transplant may reduce reinfection of the liver graft. The latter encouraging results require verification in larger trials.

When hepatitis C recurs, patients usually don't have symptoms and doctors detect it as an increase in blood levels of liver enzymes as early as one week after the transplant. Recurrent hepatitis C is often confused with rejection since the histologic features of rejection and hepatitis C on liver biopsies overlap considerably. Often, one must treat the patient based upon clinical impression and experience.

Most patients with recurrent hepatitis C do well. Only three of our patients transplanted for hepatitis C have been treated with interferon. Two of them responded with normalized liver enzymes; they remain on long-term therapy and show no progression in their liver disease. Other centers have reported that only 10 to 30 percent respond to interferon therapy.

Psychological Transformation. Post-transplant patients go through a period of accepting the "gift of life." The feelings are common to everyone and include curiosity about the donor, feelings of guilt that someone had to die so they could live, and a sense of indebtedness—of feeling overwhelmed and struggling with how to repay an enormous gift.

Michael Talamantes, transplant social worker at the University of Colorado Health Sciences Center, says that patients often write a letter of thanks to the donor's family. The donor's identity is kept confidential, so the letter is sent through official channels. If the donor's family members wish to reply, they will. And if not, it's important to respect their privacy.

Feelings of guilt over the donor's death take time to work through. Although it seems obvious that the donor's death is independent of your need for a liver, the feelings are almost universal.

> *I'm small, so I got a liver from a young boy. It blew my mind. What happened to that young man that he passed away? He was only 16 years old, still a baby. It makes me feel bad because I've been through it all.*
>
> *At first I got depressed. Then I thought maybe that's why I'm doing so well—because I've got a young, healthy liver. Finally, I said, the Lord must have wanted it this way. When I get better, I'll write to his parents . . ..*
>
> Tomas

The sense of indebtedness is often overwhelming. Some people do community service or visit patients in the hospital who are awaiting transplants. Every patient is touched in some way.

> *When I got the call for my liver, my heart went down to my toes. I was really scared. I went into the hospital restroom and confessed all my sins, restored my soul.*
>
> *Afterwards, when I recovered, I thought how beautiful the trees looked and how beautiful even the weeds looked. I went back to that restroom and thanked the Lord.*
>
> Tomas

As in every new experience, you may have contradictory feelings. It's important to pay attention to them.

Everyone talks about the "gift of life." I don't feel that way. To me, $300,000 doesn't qualify as a gift!

Sonya

It's a gift. It's unfortunate that the donor had to die, but I'm not the cause of it. Before I knew I would need a transplant, I put on my license I was a donor. I made the same decision, and I honor my donor's decision.

Sandy

Whatever normal, contradictory feelings you have, you need to sort through them to adjust to your new sense of yourself. To complicate matters, you may get mixed messages from others. Are you a hero, a biotechnological miracle, or does your boss see you as damaged goods, a drain on the company's health insurance? Whatever your experiences, they are profound indeed. You are not alone in wrestling with these issues.

People who haven't had a transplant don't understand. All they see is machinery and medicines. It's really important to talk. If someone calls me, it cheers me up to just listen, to say I was there. It can't get any better than that—to talk to someone who's been there, done that.

Evie

Improved Survival Rates

The heartening news is that survival rates have increased due to advances in immunosuppression (beginning with cyclosporine in 1979) and the team approach to liver transplantation. Before cyclosporine, patients were treated with high doses of prednisone and azathioprine. Procedures, such as thoracic duct drainage, splenectomy, and anti-lymphocyte immunoglobulin injections, were used to further suppress the immune system and prevent rejection. Before 1979, results were poor: 32 percent of patients survived one year and only 22 percent survived 30 months.

FIGURE 9. LIVER TRANSPLANT SURVIVAL RATES IN COLORADO, UNITED STATES, AND EUROPE , 1988 TO 1995.

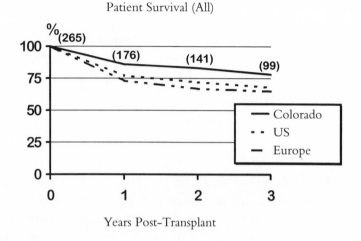

Patient Survival (All)

Years Post–Transplant

The picture has changed dramatically. Current liver transplant results show that average one- and three-year patient survival rates in the U.S. from 1988 to 1995 were 77 and 68 percent respectively. During the same period the average one- and three-year survival rates in Europe were 73 and 65 percent. Our results at the University of Colorado compared favorably to the overall results in both the U.S. and Europe: one and three-year patient survival rates were 86 and 78 percent (see Figure 9).

The reality is, however, that not all patients survive. Deaths occurring within the first six months are due to nonfunction of the donor's liver, clotting of the main artery to the liver, infection, multi-organ failure, or rejection. When deaths occur later after the transplant, they are more commonly due to malignancy or complications of atherosclerosis and rarely to rejection or infection.

The outlook is very hopeful. We anticipate that current immunosuppressive protocols will reduce adverse metabolic effects and continue to improve the long-term outlook for transplant recipients. (Since 1995 one-year survival rates at the University of Colorado exceed 90 percent.) Our ultimate goal, of course, is to restore you to your normal life.

How Organs Are Allocated

UNOS. In the United States, the United Network for Organ-Sharing (UNOS) regulates the distribution or allocation of donor organs. Here's how it works.

The United States is divided into 11 regions for organ procurement and allocation. Several local organ procurement organizations (OPOs) exist within each region. When a patient is approved for transplantation, he or she is placed on local, regional, and national waiting lists. Typically, more than 80 percent of recipients receive organs from local donors.

As waiting lists continue to expand, will a shortage of donors lead to increasing numbers of people dying while they wait for a liver? Although the number of patients listed more than tripled from 1988 to 1995—and the number of liver transplants only doubled—the waiting list mortality rate of approximately 8 percent did not change. Two factors have kept the waiting list mortality constant: earlier listing and transplantation at more urgent UNOS status.

The shortage of donors, however, has prompted certain centers to propose that one national list of recipients be formed and all donor livers in the country be allocated based upon this list. The proposal has significant drawbacks:

- Local donor organs may not serve their own community.
- Organs shipped great distances will experience more damage, reducing quality and perhaps increasing the re-transplant rate.
- If only the sickest patients are transplanted, overall patient outcomes will be poorer.
- Transportation costs will increase the cost of the transplant.
- Most centers feel that the current system is relatively fair and equitable with one exception. A regional system is needed to obtain organs quickly for the most seriously ill patients, and such plans are currently undergoing evaluation and implementation.

Centers of Excellence. UNOS publishes the results from each liver transplantation program in the United States. Patient and graft survivals are catalogued for one- and three-year outcomes. Results are also adjusted for differences in patient populations according to variables known to influence outcome after liver transplantation: UNOS listing status, diagnosis of fulminant hepatic failure, age, renal failure, presence of hepatitis B, and presence of primary liver cancer. Using this stratification method, results from each center can be compared to the expected outcome.

Intuitively, one could suggest that this analysis identifies true "centers of excellence," because it is based solely upon adjusted medical outcomes. Unfortunately, this criteria has not surfaced as the most relevant factor when negotiating contracts with third-party insurers.

Medicare was the first to put into practice the concept of centers of excellence in liver transplantation. Additional third-party insurers, such as Blue Cross/Blue Shield, Prudential, United Resource Network, and others, followed suit with similar criteria. Kaiser-Permanente also had similar guidelines, but now uses cost containment as a key factor when contracting for transplant services. With the explosion of HMOs the criteria for designating centers of excellence became even more of a mixture of medical outcome and economic impact. In some cases, it would appear that the main criteria for becoming a transplant center for a given third-party payor is simply to offer the lowest price.

Many people have suggested that the current number of 117 transplant programs is far in excess of what the donor organ pool can provide. They feel that the actual number of programs should be closer to 50 or 60. In fact, nearly half the programs in the U.S. perform fewer than 20 liver transplants per year; 75 percent of all liver transplants are performed by only 25 percent of the programs.

Several studies confirm that transplant teams with more than a minimal activity of 20 transplants per year achieve optimal patient and graft survival. Half the programs in the U.S. fall below this level of activity, further questioning the wisdom of the current proliferation of centers.

Some states have invoked the concept of "certification of need" to ensure a balance between the regional need for transplantation and the number of transplant centers. Further increases in the number of transplant centers should be discouraged unless dictated by regional requirements.

Resource: Call the toll-free UNOS patient information number at 1-888-TXINFO1 (1-888-894-6361).

Resource: To request free single copies of the following brochures, write to UNOS, P.O. Box 13770, Richmond, VA 23225: *What Every Patient Needs to Know; Questions Patients Should Ask; Share Your Life...Share Your Decision*SM*; Financing Transplantation: What Every Patient Needs to Know (3rd Edition); Questions and Answers (Spanish edition available); Did You Know?*

Resource: The *1994 Report of Center Specific Graft and Patient Survival Rates* is a listing of actual and expected outcomes by individual transplant centers for all transplants occurring between October 1, 1987 and December 31, 1989. Data on up to 10 individual transplant programs, along with a user's guide to the report, may be obtained free of charge by sending a written request to the UNOS Communications Department, P.O. Box 13770, Richmond, VA 23225, or by fax to 804-330-8507. To order an entire set of data or a volume listing all centers by one organ type (for example, data for all liver programs), contact the UNOS Professional Services Department at 804-330-8541 for price and availability.

Resource: UNOS World Wide Web site for general information on transplants, including *Data Highlights from the 1996 Annual Report*: http:\\www.unos.org.

Resource: Regional organ recovery organizations are a good source of information. For example, in Colorado and for most of Wyoming call the Colorado Organ Recovery Systems, Inc.: 303-321-0060 or 1-800-448-4644. If you don't know how to locate your region's organization, call the UNOS patient information number listed above.

Resource: You may also request the free brochure entitled *Share Your Life . . . Share Your Decision*SM*, from the Coalition on Donation: 1-800-355-SHARE.

Resource: For a free *Transplant Support Group Directory* (of more than 400 pre- and post-transplant support groups nation-wide) and a sample copy of the *Encore* newsletter (dedicated to organ transplantation), call Chronimed Pharmacy: 1-800-888-5753 and ask for a patient specialist.

Resource: For free pamphlets and information about transplants and organ donation, call a nationwide support group for transplant patients and their families, Transplant Recipients International Organization (TRIO): 1-800-TRIO-386.

> *To every thing there is a season, and a time to every purpose under the heaven. . .*
>
> *A time to weep, and a time to laugh; a time to mourn, and a time to dance. . .*
>
> Ecclesiastes

10

Research Trends
Hope for the Future

Although I try to anchor myself in the present and enjoy life day by day, I spend a lot of time worrying about the future. Will researchers perfect a protease inhibitor soon enough to help me? Will they come up with a technique that can keep a person with liver disease alive, like dialysis for patients with kidney failure?

At my support group, we announce each tiny advance and permit ourselves the necessity of hope. The future looks promising, but we know that hepatitis C doesn't get much press, and that we need lots more money spent on research.

Here's where we can do something. Each of us can talk about hepatitis C and increase awareness. Each of us can contribute time and money to finding the cure.

It's scary to know that a virus is circulating in your body, and that you can't get rid of it. Interferon works for a few people—some 10 to 30 percent—but all of us feel that there's got to be something better coming down the pike. And we wait and hope.

Hedy

A S   A   H E P A T O L O G I S T dealing with hepatitis C, I find it frustrating not to have more tools to treat my patients. Antiviral research is in its pioneer stage. I look forward to the next few years, and I expect to see exciting new advances.

Hepatitis C research falls into two broad and somewhat overlapping categories: clinical research and basic research. Clinical research primarily determines whether new drug therapies are effective in treating hepatitis C. Basic research encompasses a wide variety of studies of hepatitis C, including, but not limited to: molecular biology, cell biology, cryobiology and liver cell transplantation, pathophysiology, and pharmacology.

In this final chapter, we'll cover the following topics:

- Clinical Research: Testing New Drugs
    Phases of Clinical Trials
    Should You Sign Up for a Study?
- Current Clinical Research for Treatment of Hepatitis C
    Thymosin
    Ribavirin
    Amantadine
    Interferon Plus Ribavirin
    Long-Acting Interferons
- Potential New Therapies
    Vaccine Development
    Protease Inhibitors
    Gene Therapy
- Basic Research
    Molecular Virology
    Cell Biology
    Cryobiology and Liver Cell Transplantation
    Pathophysiology
    Pharmacology
    The Bioartificial Liver
- Research Funding

Clinical Research: Testing New Drugs

In the United States pharmaceutical companies, the National Institutes of Health, and some large universities test promising new drugs and submit their results to the Food and Drug Administration (FDA). It is the responsibility of the FDA to critically examine the results of the studies and determine whether the new treatment is safe and effective through a careful system of checks and balances. State review boards also monitor studies and adverse reactions to medications. Drugs approved by the FDA become available to practicing physicians to use in the treatment of hepatitis C.

A well-defined process evaluates all new drugs. First, the drug's safety must be established through animal testing. These studies may also help to define the expected effectiveness and dose ranges of the drug when it is used later in humans. After a drug has undergone animal testing and has been approved by the FDA for clinical research with humans, the drug testing enters three phases.

Phases of Clinical Trials. Studies in Phase I (human toxicity) typically involve small numbers of patients or healthy controls who are given single doses of the drug in varying amounts. Patients are monitored very closely (physical examinations and blood testing) to detect any adverse effect of the medication. Researchers examine the absorption of the drug, its distribution in the body, metabolism, and elimination. Sometimes the cumulative toxicity of multiple doses of drug are examined in Phase I studies.

Phase II (dose finding) studies evaluate the response of the disease to the drug in large numbers of study subjects. Researchers determine the effectiveness of several different doses of the drug administered over prolonged periods of time to find the "optimal dose" for use in humans. Patients are also carefully monitored for evidence of toxicity.

Phase III (pre-clinical testing) typically treats hundreds to thousands of patients. Again, effectiveness and toxicity are carefully evaluated. Researchers often compare the drug under investigation to existing therapies and medications to obtain a measure of whether the new treatment represents an advance above current treatment strategies. These are the final studies done to obtain FDA approval and will determine how the drug is labeled. After this phase is completed, the results are submitted to the FDA for review. Although some drugs, such as those to treat cancer, AIDS, and ALS, are on a fast track for FDA approval, it may take approximately two years for other drugs to be approved. The FDA may approve the drug, reject it, or request more studies.

Ongoing clinical testing (post-marketing surveillance for problems that might arise) occurs after the FDA has approved the drug, usually for the first one to two years, and determines optimal ways to use the drug or new indications for using the drug.

Should You Sign Up for a Study? Obviously, before you enroll in a specific study, you should take time to review the patient informed consent document that you will have to sign. Be sure to ask how often you will see a doctor; doctor appointments vary at different study sites. You also should consider all the pros and cons of any study.

On the positive side:

1. You may get to try a new treatment that is not available through general clinical practice.
2. Typically, you would receive frequent examinations and careful follow-up.
3. Study coordinators will keep you informed about your status and progress.
4. Most studies are sponsored by either pharmaceutical companies or research grants, and typically your treatment is delivered without expense to you or your insurer. However, the degree of compensation can vary and you (or your insurer) may be responsible for some of the bill. Some studies also give extra compensation to you for expenses related to travel to the study site or for the time you spent participating in the research.
5. Your participation is kept confidential. Representatives from the FDA or study sponsors, however, have the right to review your study record.
6. You reserve the right to stop treatment and withdraw from the study at any time.

On the negative side:

1. Testing programs are rigid. You must make the time commitment to follow the protocol exactly. For example, you'll have to show up at certain times for follow-up tests.
2. Clinical trials are usually blinded. That means that you won't know what you're getting in terms of dosage or placebo, for example. If you have been given a placebo, the pharmaceutical company may offer the active drug to you (free of charge) at the end of your participation in the trial if you completed the study.
3. Sponsors can stop the trials at any time.
4. You may experience undocumented side effects.
5. You must be prepared to reveal all aspects of your physical and emotional health.
6. You won't know the results of the whole study, or your individual results, until every participant has completed the protocol. It may take more than a year from your point of enrollment.

If you fail to meet criteria for entry into the controlled studies, it is still possible to be treated with investigational drugs through compassionate-use protocols. Typically, drugs available on a compassionate-use basis have been proven to be effective but have not yet received FDA approval. Physicians gain access to these drugs by contacting the pharmaceutical sponsor.

Current Clinical Research for Treatment of Hepatitis C

Optimum therapy for hepatitis C is under constant evaluation and reappraisal. One of the most exciting—and frustrating—parts of writing about clinical research is that by the time you read this chapter, researchers will be studying new treatments. At the time of this writing, however, the following drugs are under investigation.

Thymosin. Thymosin, used alone, is ineffective in eradicating hepatitis C. One trial is now comparing the effectiveness of the combination of thymosin plus interferon against interferon alone. Early analysis has suggested that the combination may be a somewhat more potent antiviral therapy than interferon alone, because patients treated with the combination have lower levels of hepatitis C virus in their blood during treatment. In addition, more of the patients on combination therapy had a complete response (normal ALT) at end of treatment. However, relapse rates were high in both groups during a six-month period of follow-up after the end of treatment.

Ribavirin. Initial studies of the use of ribavirin in the treatment of hepatitis C indicated that the drug, a nucleoside analogue, reduces the levels of ALT in blood. Despite the ability of ribavirin to lower ALT when given alone, it does not lower the blood levels of hepatitis C virus and when the drug is stopped, the ALT in all patients returns to pretreatment levels. Given this experience, ribavirin is not recommended as a single-agent therapy for patients with hepatitis C.

Amantadine. Only one study has examined the effect of amantadine in treating patients with hepatitis C. Twenty of 22 patients who had failed a previous course of interferon completed a six-month course of 200 milligrams per day of amantadine, orally. Thirty percent normalized their ALT and six out of 20 lost the hepatitis C virus from plasma by the end of the treatment period. No data on the rate of relapse was given. Additional studies are needed to determine whether amantadine should play a role in the therapy of hepatitis C.

Interferon plus Ribavirin. The reduction in ALT in patients treated with ribavirin prompted some investigators to explore the possibility that ribavirin in combination with interferon might improve the overall response to the latter treatment. Preliminary results from small trials suggest that this combination increases the likelihood of sustaining a complete response when compared to interferon alone (see Figure 10A).

In one study, groups of 15 patients (all naive to interferon therapy) were treated either with interferon alone or the combination. The complete response at end of treatment was similar between the two groups (interferon vs. combination: 80 percent vs. 73 percent for ALT and 67 percent vs. 67 percent for HCV-

FIGURE 10A. RESULTS OF COMBINATION THERAPY
WITH INTERFERON PLUS RIBAVIRIN.

Results with Interferon & Ribavirin
(Initial Experience in Small Studies)

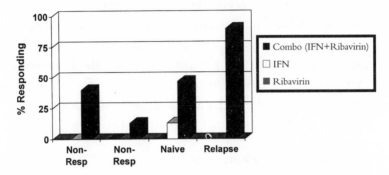

LEGEND 10A: At the time of this writing there were only a few small studies of the effectiveness of combination therapy (interferon plus ribavirin) in treating hepatitis C. In naive patients the combination was more effective in sustaining a complete response. Thirteen to 40 percent of nonresponders to interferon monotherapy were rendered ALT-normal and RNA-negative by combination therapy. Complete responders who subsequently relapse may achieve the greatest benefit from combination therapy as nearly all appear to remain ALT-normal and RNA-negative. Large multinational trials are currently underway to determine if the results from these small studies can be reproduced in greater populations of patients.

RNA). In contrast, the sustained complete response was much greater in the group treated with the combination (interferon vs. combination: 13 percent vs. 47 percent).

In addition, the combination also appears to be effective in patients who have had a complete response during interferon therapy but who relapsed once interferon was discontinued. In one trial of ten relapsed patients, nearly all patients achieved a complete response (normal ALT) by the end of treatment. Unlike other treatment studies, nearly all patients sustained their response (normal ALT 100 percent; negative HCV-RNA 90 percent). Currently, there are several trials of the use of this combination in the treatment of hepatitis C involving hundreds of patients in the United States and Europe.

Long-Acting Interferons. Several pharmaceutical companies are developing methods to modify the parent interferon molecule in order to retain antiviral activity yet deliver the active drug more slowly to the body—much like a time-release capsule. Advantages include maintaining a constant and prolonged antiviral effect and reducing the amount of injections needed. Instead of three times a week for regular interferon, the long-acting forms may need only weekly or biweekly injections. In addition, the persistent and prolonged antiviral activity afforded by these agents may aid in overall clearance of the hepatitis C virus.

Potential New Therapies

Vaccine Development. To date, researchers have made only partial and slow progress toward the development of a vaccine against hepatitis C. When vaccines were developed for hepatitis B, researchers knew that antibodies against a specific hepatitis B antigen protected against subsequent infection with hepatitis B.

Unfortunately, no naturally occurring protective antibodies have been identified for hepatitis C; all of the antibodies that have been identified do not protect against subsequent infection with hepatitis C. In addition, hepatitis C is genetically diverse, which makes it difficult to develop a single vaccine effective against all forms of the virus. Nonetheless, some advances have been made, and work is in progress.

Protease Inhibitors. Recently, a key viral enzyme has been identified, isolated, and crystallized: the HCV protease. The HCV protease is responsible for converting the large HCV protein into smaller proteins that are necessary for formation of viral particles. This protease is essential for hepatitis C to complete its life cycle. For this reason, drugs or chemicals that inactivate HCV protease would markedly inhibit viral assembly and secretion. At the time of this writing a number of pharmaceutical firms are using the crystallographic data to design specific HCV protease inhibitors.

Gene Therapy. As we learn more about the processes involved with viral replication and hepatocyte infection (cell biology) we may be able to construct biologic systems for clearing the virus from the cell. An example of this novel approach was recently published by Wu and colleagues.

These investigators were able to introduce a gene into cultured liver cells that produced an RNA that specifically inactivated hepatitis C. This RNA attached to a region in the hepatitis genes responsible for producing viral proteins. As a result, the production of viral proteins was markedly inhibited and viral replication ceased.

Obviously, this form of therapy is several years from clinical application. However, these early results suggest that gene therapy may be on the horizon as a potentially effective approach for hepatitis C.

Basic Research

Molecular Virology. Researchers have made amazing advances in understanding the hepatitis C virus, in large part because of techniques available through the new scientific field of molecular biology. As a result, scientists have completely defined the genetic makeup of the hepatitis C virus. Despite these advances, however, we still lack basic information about the proteins produced by this virus and how these proteins interact with one another and with the host cell.

Current studies are evaluating the types and properties of the proteins produced by the hepatitis C genes. It is likely that these studies will unlock the mechanisms of viral protein assembly, viral formation, and secretion of the virus out of the liver cell into blood. Understanding these critical steps required to maintain the hepatitis C infection will allow scientists to develop medications or strategies to stop the virus from reproducing (replicating) and, ultimately, to eradicate the infection.

Additional studies are trying to define how the hepatitis C virus genes control and regulate the virus's production of proteins and allow the virus to copy its own genes to make new virus. Replication maintains the infection; without it, hepatitis C would disappear after a period of time. Scientists, therefore, are looking for keys to designing drugs that will stop viral replication.

One current area of development is the HCV-specific protease inhibitors. As of this writing, none are in clinical trials. However, protease inhibitors are under development, and we anticipate that many will be tested in humans by the end of this decade. These inhibitors will inactivate the protease necessary for creating the molecules that form viral particles that are secreted from the liver cell and then reinfect adjacent cells. It is likely that protease inhibitors and other "designer" drugs will have a major impact on the treatment of hepatitis C.

Cell Biology. Despite what we do know about the hepatitis C genes and many of the proteins produced, little is known about the interaction between the hepatitis C virus and the liver cell. Future studies in this area should yield fruitful information for designing therapies, but right now many questions remain unanswered, including the following:

- What attracts hepatitis C to the liver and not to other tissues?
- How does hepatitis C bind to the surface of a liver cell and get into it?
- Once hepatitis C enters the liver cell, how does it survive?
- Why doesn't the liver cell simply swallow it up and digest it?
- What cellular systems in the liver cell are required to aid the replication of the virus?
- What are the key determinants of assembly of the viral proteins and genes to form an active infectious particle?
- What processes within the liver cell control the secretion of the viral particle out of the cell?

Cryobiology and Liver Cell Transplantation. An emerging field that is extremely exciting for both research applications and potential therapies is the isolation, storage, and subsequent use of human liver cells. These techniques have only recently become available with the development of human liver cell banks.

Dr. Bahri Bilir directs the human liver cell bank at the University of Colorado. He has managed to freeze and store (cryopreserve) human liver cells taken from several specimens of human livers recovered for use in organ transplantation but rejected due to fatty change or physical damage to the organ. After sterile preparation, cells are stored in a specialized cryopreservation medium for later thawing and use. Thawed cells are subsequently infused into patients with acute fulminant liver failure. In some cases, this technique has been successful at reversing some of the complications of liver failure and temporarily sustaining life.

Despite these initial promising results, in no case has liver cell transplantation saved patients independent of liver transplantation. Nonetheless, human liver cells have many major potential useful research applications, especially for studying the molecular virology and cell biology of hepatitis C. It is anticipated that researchers will be able to define the entire life cycle of hepatitis C with appropriate experiments using these cells.

Pathophysiology. One interesting feature of hepatitis C (and viral hepatitis in general) is that the hepatitis C infection probably is not sufficient to destroy or damage liver cells by itself. We don't fully understand the complex process of liver cell injury and the formation of fibrous tissue in the liver. Finally, repair mechanisms, such as liver regeneration, are poorly defined.

Many different laboratories are studying the effects of cofactors that may contribute to liver cell injury, fibrosis, regeneration, and progression to cirrhosis. These cofactors include processes such as excessive iron accumulation, oxidative stress, abnormal bile salts, and inflammatory mediators released by immune cells.

In the absence of effective therapies to eradicate hepatitis C, therapies that can modify basic mechanisms of cell injury and fibrosis may reduce the rate of progression to cirrhosis and the need for liver transplantation, slow the progression to liver failure, and reduce the rate of death from liver disease.

Pharmacology. As you can see, it's easy to understand that future treatment of hepatitis C could involve medications that target many different sites. I've briefly mentioned protease inhibitors, which directly target the virus. Antiviral agents that interfere with the assembly or secretions of viral genes or proteins may soon be developed.

In the absence of effective antiviral agents, treatments could focus on the mechanisms of liver cell injury. Antioxidants might be used to reduce the risk of oxidative liver cell injury. Iron removal by phlebotomy (drawing blood) may reduce storage of iron within the liver, perhaps reducing liver cell injury. Specific drugs may be developed to inhibit liver fibrosis. Undoubtedly, numerous other points of attack will be defined as our knowledge expands in the fields of molecular virology, cell biology, and pathophysiology of chronic hepatitis C.

The Bioartificial Liver. Patients who suffer from chronic kidney failure have an option, short of transplantation, that prolongs life: dialysis. Unfortunately, patients with chronic liver disease do not have a comparable liver dialysis machine.

Recently, several laboratories have begun to examine the effectiveness of bioartificial livers. Like dialysis machines, the patient's blood is passed through a capillary system to filter and cleanse the blood. The difference between standard dialysis and bioartificial livers is that liver cells are inserted into the capillary system.

The liver cells may be necessary to make the system function more like a normal liver. Theoretically, these functioning liver cells should help detoxify the patient's blood. In addition, researchers have suggested that substances synthesized and secreted by the liver cells may gain entry back into the blood and further support the patient.

Conceptually, many of the aspects of the bioartificial liver machine are sound and make sense. On the other hand, many technical problems limit the success of these machines. In the first place, the liver cells survive for only a short period of time, and cartridges need to be replaced frequently. Second, the cost of performing the dialysis is excessive. Third, the capillary barrier between plasma and liver cells is great and does not duplicate the processes of exchange between normal blood and liver cells in the patient. Fourth, none of the bioartificial liver machines have conclusively altered the outcome of patients with either chronic or acute liver failure. Thus, as of this writing, bioartificial liver machines are still considered highly experimental and unproven therapies for management of patients with liver failure.

Research Funding

It is my hope that we are entering a new era in the treatment of hepatitis C, where research may ultimately lead to discoveries of more effective treatments that benefit patients. Research into the basic mechanisms of hepatitis C replication and infection of the liver cell is absolutely essential, so that our understanding and treatment of this devastating disease may leap forward.

However, research funding for hepatitis C—although improving—is still minimal. The two agencies of the National Institutes of Health (NIH) responsible for most viral hepatitis research are the National Institute of Diabetes & Digestive & Kidney Diseases (NIDDK) and the National Institute of Allergy and Infectious Disease (NIAID). Budget estimates for 1997 hepatitis C research funding at these two agencies are $1 million and $6,418,000 respectively, totaling approximately $7,418,000. With an estimated 3.9 million people infected with hepatitis C, that's an expenditure of only $2 per patient.

Contrast that commitment to 1997 NIH research money for AIDS: a little over $1.5 billion. It's estimated that approximately 1.5 million Americans carry the HIV-AIDS virus, so research dollars total more than $1,000 per patient—about 500 times the amount spent on each person with hepatitis C.

Clearly, hepatitis C patients, friends, and family members must focus attention on research. We must make it our top priority to confront, define, and eradicate this serious viral infection, chronic hepatitis C.

Where observation is concerned,
chance favors only the prepared mind.

Louis Pasteur

Resources

Organizations

American Liver Foundation

1425 Pompton Avenue
Cedar Grove, NJ 07009-1000
1-800-GO-LIVER (465-4837)
1-888-4-HEP-ABC (443-7222)
Website: http://www.liverfoundation.org
Email: info@liverfoundation.org

Hepatitis Foundation International

30 Sunrise Terrace
Cedar Grove, NJ 07009
1-800-891-0707
Website: http://www.hepfi.org

The Hep C Connection

1741 Gaylord Street
Denver, CO 80206
303-393-9395
HepC Hotline: 1-800-522-HEPC

Hepatitis Help Line: 1-800-390-1202
Website: http://www.hepc-connection.org
Email: hepc-connection@worldnet.att.net

The Hepatitis C Foundation
1502 Russett Drive
Warminster, PA 18974
1-800-324-7305 or 215-672-2606
Website: http://www.hepcfoundation.org

Government Agencies

Centers for Disease Control and Prevention (CDC)
Hepatitis Branch, Mailstop G37
Division of Viral and Rickettsial Diseases
National Center for Infectious Diseases
Centers for Disease Control and Prevention
Atlanta, GA 30333
CDC Hepatitis Hotline: 404-332-4555
CDC Public Inquiries: 1-800-311-3435

Departments of Public Health
For information about hepatitis C in your state, call your State Department of Public Health, Epidemiology Division.

The National Institutes for Health (NIH) is the largest biomedical research center in the world. It's the research arm of the Public Health Service, U.S. Department of Health and Human Services. Among its institutes that conduct and support research on hepatitis viruses are the National Institute of Allergy and Infectious Diseases (NIAID) and the National Institute of Diabetes & Digestive & Kidney Diseases (NIDDK):

National Institute of Allergy and Infectious Diseases (NIAID)
The NIAID has the largest budget for research into viral hepatitis. In September 1996 this agency awarded four research grants

focusing on hepatitis C to four Hepatitis C Cooperative Research Centers. For an informational packet on hepatitis C, write to:

NIAID Office of Communications
Building 31
Room 7A50
Bethesda, MD 20892
301-496-5717
Press releases, fact sheets, and other materials are available on the Internet via the NIAID home page: http://www.niaid.nih.gov

National Institute of Diabetes & Digestive & Kidney Diseases (NIDDK)
For a packet of materials on hepatitis C, write to:
National Digestive Diseases Information Clearinghouse (NDDIC)
2 Information Way
Bethesda, MD 20892-3570
Website: http//www.niddk.nih.gov
Email: nddic@aerie.com

Transplant Organizations and Agencies
Transplant Recipient International Organization (TRIO)
Nationwide support group for patients and families
1735 Eye St. NW
Suite 917
Washington, DC 20006
202-293-0980

United Network for Organ Sharing (UNOS)
1100 Boulders Parkway
Suite 500
P.O. Box 13770
Richmond, VA 23225-8770
804-330-8500

Patient information: 1-888-TX INFO1 (1-888-894-6361)
Website: http://www.unos.org

U.S. Department of Health and Human Services Division of Transplantation

5600 Fishers Lane
Room 7-29
Rockville, MD 20857
301-443-7577

Note: Multiple Internet sites with information on hepatitis C exist. Although many have important information, we do not specifically endorse any of these sites and did not use any of these resources in the production of this book.

Bibliography

Chapter 1

Alter, H.J., R.H. Purcell, J.W. Shih, J.C. Melpolder, M. Houghton, Q.L. Choo, G. Kou. 1989. Detection of Antibody to Hepatitis C Virus in Prospectively Followed Transfusion Recipients with Acute and Chronic Non-A, Non-B Hepatitis. *New England Journal of Medicine*. 321:1494–1500.

Alter, M.J., H.S. Margolis, K. Krawczynski, F.N. Judson, A. Mares, W.J. Alexander, P.Y. Hu, J.K. Miller, M.A. Gerber, R.E. Sampliner, E.L. Meeks, M.J. Beach. 1992. The Natural History of Community-Acquired Hepatitis C in the United States. *New England Journal of Medicine*. 327:1899–905.

American Liver Foundation. 1995. *Getting Hip to Hep*. Cedar Grove: American Liver Foundation.

Bader, Teddy F. 1995. *Viral Hepatitis: Practical Evaluation and Treatment*. Seattle: Hogrefe & Huber.

Choo, Q.L., G. Kou, A.J. Weiner, L.R. Overby, D.W. Bradley, M. Houghton. 1989. Isolation of a cDNA Clone Derived from a Blood Borne Non-A, Non-B Viral Hepatitis Genome. *Science* 244:359–362.

Dienstag, J.L. 1990. Hepatitis Non-A, Non-B: C At Last. *Gastroenterology*. 99:1177–1180.

Kou, G., Q.L. Choo, H.J. Alter, G.L. Gitnick, A.G. Redeker, R.H. Purcell, T. Miyamura, J.L. Dienstag, M.J. Alter, C.E. Stevens, G.E. Tegtmeier, F. Bonino, M. Colombo, W.S. Lee, C. Kou, K. Berger, J.R. Shuster, L.R. Overby, D.W. Bradley, M. Houghton. 1989. An Assay for Circulating Antibodies to a Major Etiologic Virus of Human Non-A, Non-B Hepatitis. *Science*. 244:362-364.

Mandell, G.L., J.E. Bennett, R. Dolin, eds. 1995. *Principles and Practice of Infectious Diseases, Vol.2*. New York: Churchill Livingstone.

Radetsky, P. 1994. *The Invisible Invaders: Viruses and the Scientists Who Pursue Them*. Boston: Little, Brown and Co.

Shimizu, Y.K., S.M. Feinstone, M. Kohara, R.H. Purcell, H. Yoshikura. February 1996. Hepatitis C Virus: Detection of Intracellular Virus Particles by Electron Microscopy. *Hepatology*. 23:205-209.

"Hepatitis C." World Health Organization. *Weekly Epidemiological Record*. 7 March 1997: 65-69.

Chapter 2

Kato, N., O. Yokosuka, M. Omata, K. Hosoda, M. Ohto. 1990. Detection of Hepatitis C Virus Ribonucleic Acid in the Serum by Amplification with Polymerase Chain Reaction. *Journal of Clinical Investigation*. 86:1764-1767.

Lau, J.Y.N., G.L. Davis, L.E. Prescott, G. Maertens, K.L. Lindsay, K.P. Qian, M. Mizokami, P. Simmonds, and Hepatitis Interventional Therapy Group. 1996. Distribution of Hepatitis C Virus Genotypes Determined by Line Probe Assay in Patients with Chronic Hepatitis C Seen at Tertiary Referral Centers in the United States. *Annals of Internal Medicine*. 124:868-76.

McHutchison, J.G., J.L. Person, S. Govindarajan, B. Valinluck, T. Gore, S.R. Lee, M. Nelles, A. Polito, D. Chien, R. DiNello, S. Quan, G. Kuo, A.G. Redeker. 1992. Improved Detection of Hepatitis C Virus Antibodies in High-risk Populations. *Hepatology*. 15:19-25.

Ohno, T., J.Y.N. Lau. 1996. The "Gold-Standard," Accuracy, and the Current Concepts: Hepatitis C Virus Genotype and Viremia (editorial). *Hepatology*. 24:1312–1315.

Tedeschi, V., L.B. Seef. 1995. Diagnostic Tests for Hepatitis C: Where Are We Now? (editorial). *Annals of Internal Medicine*. 123:383–385.

Ulrich, P.P., J.M. Romeo, P.K. Lane, I. Kelly, L.J. Daniel, G.N. Vyas. 1990. Detection, Semiquantitation, and Genetic Variation in Hepatitis C Virus Sequences Amplified from the Plasma of Blood Donors with Elevated Alanine Aminotransferase. *Journal of Clinical Investigation*. 86:1609–1614.

Yoshioka, K., S. Kakumu, T. Wakita, T. Ishikawa, Y. Itoh, M. Takayanagi, Y. Higashi, M. Shibata, T. Morishima. 1991. Detection of Hepatitis C Virus by Polymerase Chain Reaction and Response to Interferon-α Therapy: Relationship to Genotypes of Hepatitis C Virus. *Hepatology*. 16:293–299.

Zein, N.N., J. Rakela, E. Krawitt, K.R. Reddy, T. Tominaga, D. Persing, and the Collaborative Study Group. 1996. Hepatitis C Virus Genotypes in the United States: Epidemiology, Pathogenicity, and Response to Interferon Therapy. *Annals of Internal Medicine*. 125:634–640.

Chapter 3

Bader, T.F. 1995. *Viral Hepatitis: Practical Evaluation and Treatment*. Seattle:Hogrefe & Huber. 144–150.

Benamouzig, R., V. Ezratty, S. Chaussade. 1990. Risk for Type C Hepatitis Through Sexual Contact (editorial). *Annals of Internal Medicine*. 113:638.

Castrone, L. 2 July 1996. Piercing and Tattooing, Body Language of 90s Worries Health Experts. *Rocky Mountain News*. 3D.

Donahue, J.G., A. Munoz, P.M. Ness, D.E. Brown, D.H. Yawn, H.A. McAllister, B.A. Reitz, K.E. Nelson. 1992. The Declining Risk of Post-transfusion Hepatitis C Virus Infection. *New England Journal of Medicine*. 327:369–73.

Esteban, J.I., A. González, J.M. Hernández, L. Viladomiu, C. Sánchez, J.C. López-Talavera, D. Lucea, C. Martin-Vega, X.

Vidal, R. Esteban, J. Guardia. 1990. Evaluation of Antibodies to Hepatitis C Virus in a Study of Transfusion-Associated Hepatitis. *New England Journal of Medicine.* 323:1107–1112.

Everhart, J.E., A.M. DiBisceglie, L.M. Murray, H.J. Alter, J.J. Melpolder, G. Kuo, J. Hoofnagle. 1990. Risk for Non-A, Non-B (Type C) Hepatitis Through Sexual or Household Contact with Chronic Carriers. *Annals of Internal Medicine.* 112:544–545.

Hollinger, F.B., J.L. Hsiang. 1992. Community-Acquired Hepatitis C Virus Infection (editorial). *Gastroenterology.* 102:1425–29.

Hoyos, M., J.V. Sarrión, T. Péres-Castellanos, M. Prieto, M.L. Marty, V. Garrigues, J. Berenguer. 1989. Prospective Assessment of Donor Blood Screening for Antibody to Hepatitis B Core Antigen as a Means of Preventing Posttransfusion Non-A, Non-B, Hepatitis. *Hepatology.* 9:449–451.

Keeping Score 1996. Washington: Drug Strategies, 1996.

Kelen, G.D., G.B. Green, R.H. Purcell, D.W. Chan, B.F. Qaqish, K.T. Sivertson, T.C. Quinn. 1992. Hepatitis B and Hepatitis C in Emergency Department Patients. *New England Journal of Medicine.* 326:1399–404.

Koff, R.S. 1992. The Low Efficiency of Maternal-Neonatal Transmission of Hepatitis C Virus: How Certain Are We? (editorial). *Annals of Internal Medicine.* 117:967–969.

Long, G.E., L.S. Rickman. 1994. Infectious Complications of Tattoos. *Clinical Infectious Diseases.* 18:610–9.

Mannucci, P.M., K. Schimpf, B. Brettler, N. Ciavarella, M. Colombo, F. Haschke, K. Lechner, J. Lusher, G. Weissbach, and the International Study Group. 1990. Low Risk for Hepatitis C in Hemophiliacs Given a High-Purity, Pasteurized Factor VIII Concentrate. *Annals of Internal Medicine.* 113:27–32.

McCashland, T.M., T.L. Wright, J.P. Donovan, D.F. Schafer, M.F. Sorrell, T.G. Heffron, A.N. Langnas, I.J. Fox, B.W. Shaw, Jr., R.K. Zetterman. 1995. Low Incidence of Intraspousal Transmission of Hepatitis C Virus after Liver Transplantation. *Liver Transplantation and Surgery*. 1:358-361.

Mitsui, T., K. Iwano, K. Masuko, C. Yamazaki, H. Okamoto, F. Tsuda, T. Tanaka, S. Mishiro. 1992. Hepatitis C Virus Infection in Medical Personnel After Needlestick Accident. *Hepatology*. 16:1109-1114.

Ohto, H., S. Terazawa, N. Sasaki, N. Sasaki, K. Hino, C. Ishiwata, M. Kako, N.Ujiie, C. Endo, A. Matsui, H. Okamoto, S. Mishiro, and the Vertical Transmission of Hepatitis C Virus Collaborative Study Group. 1994. Transmission of Hepatitis C Virus from Mothers to Infants. *New England Journal of Medicine*. 330:744-50.

Pereira, B.J.G., E.L. Milford, R.L. Kirkman, A.S. Levey. 1991. Transmission of Hepatitis C Virus by Organ Transplantation. *New England Journal of Medicine*. 325:454-60.

Pereira, B.J.G., E.L. Milford, R.L. Kirkman, S. Quan, K.R. Sayre, P.J. Johnson, J.C. Wilber, A.S. Levey. 1992. Prevalence of Hepatitis C Virus RNA in Organ Donors Positive for Hepatitis C Antibody and in the Recipients of Their Organs. *New England Journal of Medicine*. 327:910-5.

Roth, D., J.A. Fernandez, S. Babischkin, A. De Mattos, B.E. Buck, S. Quan, L. Olson, G.W. Burke, J.R. Nery, V. Esquenazi, E.R. Schiff, J. Miller. 1992. Detection of Hepatitis C Virus Infection among Cadaver Organ Donors: Evidence for Low Transmission of Disease. *Annals of Internal Medicine*. 117:470-475.

Roudot-Thoraval, F., J. Pawlotsky, V. Thiers, L. Deforges, P. Girollet, F. Guillot, C. Huraux, P. Aumont, C. Brechot, D. Dhumeaux. 1993. Lack of Mother-to-infant Transmission of Hepatitis C Virus in Human Immunodeficiency Virus-seronegative Women: A Prospective Study with Hepatitis C Virus RNA Testing. *Hepatology*. 17:772-777.

Rumi, M.G., M. Colombo, A. Gringeri, P.M. Mannucci. 1990. High Prevalence of Antibody to Hepatitis C Virus in Multitransfused Hemophiliacs with Normal Transaminase Levels. *Annals of Internal Medicine.* 112:379-380.

Schiff, E.R. 1992. Hepatitis C Among Health Care Providers: Risk Factors and Possible Prophylaxis (editorial). *Hepatology.* 16:1300-1301.

Schreiber, G.B., M.P. Busch, S.H. Kleinman, J.J. Korelitz, for the Retrovirus Epidemiology Donor Study. 1996. The Risk of Transfusion-Transmitted Viral Infections. *New England Journal of Medicine.* 334:1685-90.

Seeff, L.B., H.J. Alter. 1994. Spousal Transmission of the Hepatitis C Virus? (editorial). *Annals of Internal Medicine.* 120:807-809.

Seeff, L.B., Z. Buskell-Bales, E.C. Wright, S.J. Durako, H.J. Alter, F.L. Iber, F.B. Hollinger, G. Gitnick, R.G. Knodell, R.P. Perrillo, C.E. Stevens, C.G. Hollingsworth, and National Heart, Lung, and Blood Institute Study Group. 1992. Long-term Mortality after Transfusion-Associated Non-A, Non-B Hepatitis. *New England Journal of Medicine.* 327:1906-11.

Shakil, A.O., C. Conry-Cantilena, H.J. Alter, P. Hayashi, D.E. Kleiner, V. Tadeschi, K. Krawczynski, H.S. Conjeevaram, R. Sallie, A.M. Di Bisceglie, and Hepatitis C Study Group. 1995. Volunteer Blood Donors with Antibody to Hepatitis C Virus: Clinical, Biochemical, Virologic, and Histologic Features. *Annals of Internal Medicine.* 123:330-337.

Tong, M.J., N.S. El-Farra, A.R. Reikes, R.L. Co. 1995. Clinical Outcomes after Transfusion-Associated Hepatitis C. *New England Journal of Medicine.* 332:1463-6.

U.S. Department of Health and Human Services, Substance Abuse and Mental Health Services Administration. 1996. *National Household Survey on Drug Abuse: Population Estimates 1995 (Preliminary Tables).* Rockville: Office of Applied Studies.

Chapter 4

Hamilton, E. 1940, reprint 1989. *Mythology, Timeless Tales of Gods and Heroes.* Reprint. New York: Meridian.

Lyons, A.S., J.R. Petrucelli, II. 1978. *Medicine, An Illustrated History*. New York: Harry N. Abrams.

Neruda, Pablo.. 1977. *Nuevas Odas Elementales,* Cuarta Edicion. Buenos Aires; Editorial Losada.

"Sculpture in Spain Salutes the 'Silent, Unselfish' Liver." *Austin-American Statesman* 28 June 1987: A2.

Chapter 5

Caregaro, L., F. Alberino, P. Amodio, C. Merkel, M. Bolognesi, P. Angeli, A. Gatta. 1996. Malnutrition in Alcoholic and Virus-Related Cirrhosis. *American Journal of Clinical Nutrition.* 63:602-9.

Cowley, J. 6 May 1996. Herbal Warning. *Newsweek.* 63.

Munoz, S.J. 1991. Nutritional Therapies in Liver Disease. *Seminars in Liver Disease.* 11:278-291.

Nompleggi, D.J., H.L. Bonkovsky. 1994. Nutritional Supplementation in Chronic Liver Disease: An Analytical Review. *Hepatology.* 19:518-533.

U.S. Department of Agriculture, U.S. Department of Health and Human Services. 1995. *Dietary Guidelines for Americans.* Fourth Edition. Washington.

Chapter 6

Spiegel, David, M.D. 1993. *Living Beyond Limits.* New York: Random House.

Chapter 7

Beam, Jr., Burton T. and Kenn B. Tacchino. Jan. 1997. The Health Insurance Portability and Accountability Act of 1996. *Journal of the American Society of CLU & ChFC.* 14+

Health Care Financing Administration. 1996. *Your Medicare Handbook 1996.* Washington: U.S. Government Printing Office.

Jehle, F.F. 1995. *The Complete and Easy Guide to Social Security Medicare.* Peterborough: Fraser-Vance.

Social Security Administration. March 1996. *Social Security Supplemental Security Income*. SSA Publication No. 05-11000. Washington.

Social Security Administration. Feb. 1997. *Social Security Retirement Benefits*. Washington.

Social Security Administration. Sept. 1995. *Social Security Disability Programs Can Help*. SSA Publication No. 05-10057. Washington.

Social Security Administration. May 1996. *Social Security Disability Benefits*. SSA Publication No. 05-10029. Washington.

Social Security Administration. Aug. 1995. *Medicare*. Washington.

U.S. Department of Health and Human Services, Health Care Financing Administration. 1994. *Medicare and Other Health Benefits. Who Pays First?* Washington.

U.S. Department of Labor Employment Standards Administration, Wage and Hour Division. 1993. Publication 1421. *Compliance Guide to the Family and Medical Leave Act*. Washington: U.S. Government Printing Office.

U.S. Department of Labor Program. 1993. *The Family and Medical Leave Act of 1993*. Highlights Fact Sheet No. ESA 93-2. Washington: U.S. Government Printing Office.

U.S. Equal Employment Opportunity Commission, U.S. Department of Justice, Civil Rights Division. 1992. *The Americans with Disabilities Act, Questions and Answers*. Washington.

U.S. Equal Employment Opportunity Commission. 1991. *The Americans With Disabilities Act*. Washington.

United Network for Organ Sharing (UNOS) Patient Affairs Committee. *Financing Transplantation, What Every Patient Needs to Know*.

Chapter 8

Bacon, B.R., G. Farrell, J.P. Benhamou, U. Hopf, R. Barcena, V. Feinman, M. Rizzello, T. Wright, S. Warwick, J. Horton, and Wellferon Study Group. 1995. Lymphoblastoid Interferon Improves Long-term Response to a Six Month Course of

Treatment When Compared with Recombinant Interferon Alfa 2b. *Hepatology.* 22:152A.

Bonkovsky, H.L., B.F. Banner, A.L. Rothman. 1997. Iron and Chronic Viral Hepatitis. *Hepatology.* 25:759-767.

Bortolotti, F., R. Giacchino, P. Vajro, C. Barbera, C. Crivellaro, A. Alberti, G. Nebbia, L. Zancan, L. De Moliner, A. Bertolini, F. Balli, F. Callea. 1995. Recombinant Interferon-Alfa Therapy in Children with Chronic Hepatitis C. *Hepatology.* 22:1623-27.

Causse, X., H. Godinot, M. Chevallier, P. Chossegros, F. Zoulim, D. Ouzan, J.P. Heyraud, T. Fontanes, J. Albrecht, C. Meschievitz, C. Trepo. 1991. Comparison of 1 or 3 MU of Interferon Alfa-2b and Placebo in Patients with Chronic Non-A, Non-B Hepatitis. *Gastroenterology.* 101:497-502.

Chemello, L., P. Bonetti, L. Cavallettoi, F. Talato, V. Donadon, P. Casarin, F. Belussi, M. Fezza, F. Noventa, P. Pontisso, L. Benvegnu, C. Casarin, A. Alberti, the TriVeneto Viral Hepatitis Group. 1995. Randomized Trial Comparing Three Different Regimens of Alpha-2a-Interferon in Chronic Hepatitis C. *Hepatology.* 22:700-706.

Davis, G.L., L.A. Balart, E.R. Schiff, K. Lindsay, H.C. Bodenheimer, R.P. Perrillo, W. Carey, I.M. Jacobson, J. Payne, J.L. Dienstag, D.H. VanThiel, C. Tamburro, J. Lefkowitch, J. Albrecht, C. Meschievitz, T.J. Ortego, A. Gibas, and the Hepatitis Interventional Therapy Group. 1989. Treatment of Chronic Hepatitis C, with Recombinant Interferon Alfa. A Multicenter Randomized, Controlled Trial. *New England Journal of Medicine.* 321:1501-1506.

DiBisceglie, A.M., P. Martin, C. Kassianides, M. Lisker-Melman, L. Murray, J. Waggoner, Z. Goodman, S.M. Banks, J. Hoofnagle. 1989. Recombinant Interferon Alfa Therapy for Chronic Hepatitis C. A Randomized, Double-blind, Placebo-controlled Trial. *New England Journal of Medicine.* 321:1506-1510.

Diodati, G., P.K. Bonetti, F. Noventa, C. Casarin, M. Rugge, S. Scaccabarozzi, A. Tagger, L. Pollice, F. Tremolada, C. Davite,

G. Realdi, A. Ruol. 1994. Treatment of Chronic Hepatitis C with Recombinant Human Interferon-α2a: Results of a Randomized Controlled Clinical Trial. *Hepatology.* 19:1-5.

Dusheiko, G.M., J.A. Roberts. 1995. Treatment of Chronic Type B and C Hepatitis with Interferon Alfa: an Economic Appraisal. *Hepatology.* 22:1863-1873.

Hasan, F., L.J. Jeffers, M. DeMedina, K.R. Reddy, T. Parker, E.R. Schiff, M. Houghton, Q. Choo, G. Kuo. 1990. Hepatitis C-associated Hepatocellular Carcinoma. *Hepatology.* 12:589-591.

Hollinger, F.B., M.J. Tong, K.R. Reddy, W.M. Lee, P.J. Pocros, J.C. Heols, E. Keefee, J.L. Heathcote, H. White, R.T. Foust, D.M. Hensen, E.L. Krawitt, H. Fromm, M. Black, M. Klein, J. Lubina, C. Manyak, L.M. Blatt, and the Consensus Interferon Study Group Baylor College of Medicine, The Consensus Interferon Study Sites and Amgen Inc. A Phase 3 Study for the Treatment of Patients with Chronic Hepatitis C (HCV) Infection with Consensus Interferon (CIFN). Hepatology Meeting, Rome, Italy.

Hoofnagle, J.H., A.M. Di Bisceglie. 1997. The Treatment of Chronic Viral Hepatitis. *New England Journal of Medicine.* 336:347-356.

Hoofnagle, J.H., K.D. Mullen, D.B. Jones, V. Rustgi, A. DiBisceglie, M. Peters, J.G. Waggoner, Y. Park, E.A. Jones. 1986. Treatment of Chronic Non-A, Non-B Hepatitis with Recombinant Human Alpha Interferon. *New England Journal of Medicine.* 315:1575-1578.

Koff, R.S., L.B. Seeff. 1995. Economic Modeling of Treatment in Chronic Hepatitis B and Chronic Hepatitis C: Promises and Limitations. *Hepatology.* 22:1880-82.

Lampertico, P., M. Rumi, R. Romeo, A. Craxi, R. Soffredini, D. Biassoni, M. Colombo. 1994. A Multicenter Randomized Controlled Trial of Recombinant Interferon-α_{2b} in Patients with Acute Transfusion-associated Hepatitis C. *Hepatology.* 19:19-22.

Lindsay, K.L., G.L. Davis, E.R. Schiff, H.C. Bodenheimer, L.A. Balart, J.L. Dienstag, R.P. Perrillo, C.H. Tamburro, J.S. Goff, G.T. Everson, M. Silva, W.N. Katkov, Z. Goodman, J.Y.N. Lau, G. Maertens, J. Gogate, B. Sanghvi, J. Albrecht, and the Hepatitis Interventional Therapy Group. 1996. Response to Higher Doses of Interferon Alfa-2b in Patients with Chronic Hepatitis C: A Randomised Multicenter Trial. *Hepatology.* 24:1034-1040.

Marcellin, P., N. Boyer, E. Giostra, C. Degott, A.M. Courouc, F. Degos, H. Coppere, P. Cales, P.K. Couzigou, J.P. Benhamou. 1991. Recombinant Human α-Interferon in Patients with Chronic Non-A, Non-B Hepatitis: a Multicenter Randomized Controlled Trial from France. *Hepatology.* 13:393-397.

Marcellin, P., M. Pouteau, M. Martinot-Peignoux, F. Degos, V. Duchatelle, N.M. Boyer, C. Lemonnier, C. Degott, S. Erlinger, P. Benhamou. 1995. Lack of Benefit of Escalating Dosage of Interferon Alfa in Patients with Chronic Hepatitis C. *Gastroenterology.* 109:156-165.

Niederau, C., T. Heintges, D. Häussinger. 1995. Treatment of Chronic NANB and C Hepatitis with α-Interferon: A Meta-Analysis of Dose and Duration. *Hepatology.* 22 (4):153A.

Poynard, T., P. Bedossa, M. Chevallier, P. Mathurin, C. Lemonnier, C. Trepo, P. Couzigou, J.L Payen, M. Sajus, J.M. Costa, M. Vadaud, J.C. Chaput, the Multicenter Study Group. 1995. A Comparison of Three Interferon Alfa-2b Regimens for the Long-term Treatment of Chronic Non-A, Non-B Hepatitis. *New England Journal of Medicine.* 332:1457-62.

Poynard, T., V. Leroy, M. Cohard, T. Thevenot, P. Mathurin, P. Opolon, J.P. Zarski. 1996. Meta-Analysis of Interferon Randomized Trials in the Treatment of Viral Hepatitis C: Effects of Dose and Duration. *Hepatology.* 24:778-789.

Reichard, O., H. Glaumann, A. Fryden, G. Norkrans, R. Schvarcz, A. Soonerborg, Z.B. Yun, O. Weiland. 1995. Two Year Biochemical, Virological, and Histological Follow-Up in Patients with Chronic Hepatitis C Responding in a Sustained

Fashion to Interferon Alfa-2b Treatment. *Hepatology*. 21:918-922.

Ruiz-Moreno, M., M.J. Rua, I. Castillo, M.D. Garcia-Novo, M. Santos, S. Navas, V. Carreno. 1992. Treatment of Children with Chronic Hepatitis C with Recombinant Interferon-α: a Pilot Study. *Hepatology*. 16:882-885.

Rumi, M., E.D. Ninno, M.L. Parravicini, R. Romeo, R. Soffredini, M.F. Donato, J. Wilber, A. Russo, M. Colombo. 1996. A Prospective, Randomized Trial Comparing Lymphoblastoid to Recombinant Interferon Alfa 2a As Therapy for Chronic Hepatitis C. *Hepatology*. 24:1366-1370.

Saez-Royela, F., J.C. Porres, A. Moreno, I. Castillo, G. Martinez, F. Galiana, V. Carreno. 1991. High Dose of Recombinant Alpha-interferon or Gamma interferon for Chronic Hepatitis C: A Randomized, Controlled Trial. *Hepatology*. 13:327-331.

Saracco, G., F. Bosina, M.L. Abate, L. Chiandussi, V. Gallo, E. Cerutti, A. Di Napoli, A. Solinas, A. Deplano, A. Tocco, P. Cossu, D. Dhien, G. Kuo, A. Polito, A.J. Weiner, M. Houghton, G. Verme, F. Bonino, M. Rizzetto. 1993. Long-term Follow-up of Patients with Chronic Hepatitis C Treated with Different Doses of Interferon-α2b. *Hepatology*. 18:1300-1305.

Schvarcz, R., Z.B. Yun, A. Sonnerborg, O. Weiland. 1995. Combined Treatment with Interferon Alpha-2b and Ribavirin for Chronic Hepatitis C in Patients with a Previous Non-response or Non-sustained Response to Interferon Alone. *Journal of Medical Virology*. 43:43-7.

Serfaty, L., O. Chazouilleres, J.M. Pawlotsky, T. Andreani, C. Pellet, R. Poupon. 1996. Interferon Alfa Therapy in Patients with Chronic Hepatitis C and Persistently Normal Aminotransferase Activity. *Gastroenterology*. 5110:291-295.

Shiffman, M.L., C.M. Hofmann, V.A. Luketic, A.J. Sanyal, M.J. Contos, A.S. Mills. 1996. Improved Sustained Response Following Treatment of Chronic Hepatitis C by Gradual Reduction in the Interferon Dose. *Hepatology*. 24:21-26.

Simon, D.M., S.C. Gordon, M.M. Kaplan, R.S. Koff, F. Regenstein, G. Everson, Y.M. Lee, F. Weiner, A. Silverman, T. Plasse, D. Fedorczyk, M. Liao. 1997. Treatment of Chronic Hepatitis C with Interferon Alfa-n3: A Multicenter, Randomized, Open-Label Trial. *Hepatology.* 25:445-448.

Viladomiu, L., J. Genesca, J.I. Esteban, H. Allende, A. Gonzalez, J.C. Lopez-Talavera, R. Esteban, J. Guardia. 1992. Interferon-α in Acute Posttransfusion Hepatitis C: A Randomized, Controlled Trial. *Hepatology.* 15:767-769.

Woolf, G.M., L.M. Petrovic, S.E. Rojter, S. Wainwright, F.G. Villamil, W.N. Katkov, P. Michieletti, I.R. Wanless, F.R. Stermitz, J.J. Beck, J.M.Vierling. 1994. Acute Hepatitis Associated with the Chinese Herbal Product Jin Bu Huan. *Annals of Internal Medicine.* 121:729-735.

Chapter 9

Chazouilleres, O., M. Kim, C. Combs, L. Ferrell, P. Bacchetti, J. Roberts, N.L. Ascher, P. Neuwald, J. Wilber, M. Urdea, S. Quan, R. Sanchez-Pescador, T.L. Wright. 1994. Quantitation of Hepatitis C Virus RNA in Liver Transplant Recipients. *Gastroenterology.* 106:994-999.

Dienstag, J.L. 1997. The Natural History of Chronic Hepatitis C and What We Should Do About It. *Gastroenterology.* 112:651-655.

Everson, G.T., I. Kam. 1996. Liver Transplantation: Current Status and Unresolved Controversies. *Advances in Internal Medicine.* Vol. 42. London: Mosby-Year Book, Inc. pp. 505-553.

Fattovich, G., G. Giustina, F. Degos, F. Tremolada, G. Diodati, P. Almasio, F. Nevens, A. Solinas, D. Mura, J.T. Brouwer, H. Thomas, C. Njapoum, C. Casarin, P. Bonetti, P. Fuschi, J. Basho, A. Tocco, A. Bhalla, R. Galassini, F. Noventa, S.W. Schalm, G. Realdi. 1997. Morbidity and Mortality in Compensated Cirrhosis Type C: A Retrospective Follow-up Study of 384 Patients. *Gastroenterology.* 112:463-472.

Ferrell, L.D., T.L. Wright, J. Roberts, N. Ascher, J. Lake. 1992. Hepatitis C Viral Infection in Liver Transplant Recipients. *Hepatology.* 16:865–876.

Gane, E.J., N.V. Naoumov, K.P. Qian, M.U. Mondelli, G. Maertens, B.C. Portmann, J.Y.N. Lau, R. Williams. 1996. A Longitudinal Analysis of Hepatitis C Virus Replication Following Liver Transplantation. *Gastroenterology.* 110:167–177.

Gane, E.J., B.C. Portmann, N. Naoumov, H.M. Smith, J.A. Underhill, P.T. Donaldson, G. Maertens, R. Williams. 1996. Long-term Outcome of Hepatitis C Infection after Liver Transplantation. *New England Journal of Medicine.* 334:815–20.

Chapter 10

Brillanti, S., J. Garson, M. Foli, K. Whitby, R. Deaville, C. Masi, M. Miglioli, L. Barbara. 1994. A Pilot Study of Combination Therapy with Ribavirin Plus Interferon Alfa for Interferon Alfa Resistant Chronic Hepatitis C. *Gastroenterology.* 107:812–7.

Brouwer, J.T., F. Nevens, P. Michielsen, M.L. Hautekeete, R.A.F.M. Chamuleau, M. Adler, et al. 1994. What Options Are Left When Hepatitis C Does Not Respond to Interferon? Placebo-controlled Benelux Multicenter Retreatment Trial on Ribavrin Monotherapy Versus Combination with Interferon. *Journal of Hepatology.* 21(Suppl. 1):S17.

Chemello, L., L. Cavalletto, E. Bernardinello, E. Suivlestri, L. Benveganu, P. Pontisso, et al. 1994. Response to Ribavirin, to Interferon and to a Combination of Both in Patients with Chronic Hepatitis C and its Relation to HCV Genotypes. *Journal of Hepatology.* 21(Suppl. 1):12.

Department of Health and Human Services, Food and Drug Administration. March 1990. *From Test Tube to Patient: New Drug Development in the United States.* An FDA Consumer Special Report, DHHS Publication No. 90-3168. Rockville: Jan. 1988, Rev.

Di Bisceglie, A.M., H.S. Conjeevaram, M.W. Fried, R. Sallie, Y. Park, C. Yurdaydin, M. Swain, D.E. Kleiner, K. Mahaney,

J.H. Hoofnagle. 1995. Ribavirin as Therapy for Chronic Hepatitis C, A Randomized, Double-Blind, Placebo-Controlled Trial. *Annals of Internal Medicine*. 123:897-903.

Lai, M. Y., J.H. Kao, P.M. Yang, J.T. Wang, P.J. Chen, K.W. Chan, J.S. Chu, D.S. Chen. 1996. Long-term Efficacy of Ribavirin Plus Interferon Alfa in the Treatment of Chronic Hepatitis C. *Gastroenterology*. 111:1307-1312.

Rasi, G., M.G. Mutchnick, D. DiVirgilio, P. Pierimarchi, P. Sinibaldi-Vallebona, F. Colella, E. Garaci. 1995. Combination Thymosin α1 (Tα1) and Lymphoblastoid Interferon (L-IFN) Therapy in Chronic Hepatitis C (CHC). *Gastroenterology*. 108(4): A1153.

Rezakovic, I., C. Zavaglia, R. Bottelli, G. Idéo. 1993. A Pilot Study of Thymosin Alpha 1 Therapy in Chronic Active Hepatitis C. *Hepatology*. 18(4):252A.

Sakamoto, N., C.H. Wu, G.Y. Wu. 1996. Intracellular Cleavage of Hepatitis C Virus RNA and Inhibition of Viral Protein Translation by Hammerhead Ribozymes. *Journal of Clinical Investigation*. 98:2720-8.

Sarnow, P. 1995. *Current Topics in Microbiology and Immunology*. Volume 203; Berlin Heidelberg: Springer-Verlag. pp: 99-112.

Smith, J.P. 1996. Treatment of Chronic Hepatitis C with Amantadine Hydrochloride. *Gastroenteology*. 110(4):A1330.

Index

THE SECRET STRENGTH OF DEPRESSION
by Frederic Flach, MD

'Turn depression into expression –
and gain new energy zest, and self-respect..."
– *The Denver Post*

The Secret Strength of Depression, first published in 1974, has been acclaimed as one of the clearest and most helpful books available on the subject of depression.

Now fully revised and updated for the 1990s, this new presentation incorporates the latest discoveries in the treatment of depression, including new approaches to psychotherapy and the myths and miracles of the new antidepressants.

Depression is a normal healthy process, according to Dr. Flach. It stimulates the process of learning and change, and often accompanies major life cycle transitions: graduating from school, getting married, retirement, the loss of a loved one. Depression only becomes an illness when its severity cannot be contained, when a person isn't equipped to handle its pain or its perceived shame, or when it persists for too long a time, often for years after the stressful events that have given rise to it.

Overcoming depression and learning from it is an invaluable source of strength and growth. This positive attitude has made dealing with depression and the process of treatment for it much easier for many thousands of people ... The Secret Strength goes a long way toward destigmatizing depression and encouraging people to take the necessary first steps to recover.

"... There should be a considerable readership for this informed, hopeful, and helpful look at the malaise in layman's terms.. Dr. Flach's credentials lend weight to his views and insights... "

–Publishers Weekly

Dr. Flach is Adjunct Associate Professor of Psychiatry at Cornell University Medical College Attending Psychiatrist at both the New York Hospital-Cornell Medical Center and Saint Vincent's Hospital and Medical Center of New York His central interests have focused on the subjects of depression and stress management for 30 years. His books have included *A New Marriage, A New Life;* and the bestsellers *Resilience* and *Rickie*. He has been a guest an many national television broadcasts, including *Good Morning America, The Today Show,* and *Donohue!*

PRICE	PAGES	ISBN	CATEGORY
$14.95 Pbk	272	1-886330-02-6	Psychology/Health/Self-help

Available at bookstores everywhere or direct from the publisher at
1-800-906-1234.
Visit our health and self-help website www.takecommand.com

WOMEN and ANXIETY
REVISED EDITION
A Step-by-Step Program for Managing Anxiety and Depression
by Helen A. DeRosis, M.D.

Anxiety and Depression are Facts of Life, but You Don't Have to Live with Them!

Single parenthood. Marriage problems. AIDS. Sexual freedom. Divorce. Career demands. The glass ceiling. Run with the Wolves or play by The Rules. Pro-life. Choice. Alternative lifestyles.

NO WONDER women are anxious and depressed. Never before have women been confronted with so many bewildering choices and so many incessant demands. How do women cope? How can they defeat self-defeating attitudes and actions? How can they conquer their fears, win the battle with anxiety and triumph over depression?

Women and Anxiety, first published in 1979, has been hailed as a book that "every woman-married, single, working, or home-oriented-could use to help her live a fuller, free-of -fear life." Now completely revised and updated for the 1990s, *Women and Anxiety* offers readers a new, dynamic, and easy-to-use strategy for dealing with the problems of stress, anxiety, and depression. In an inspiring and practical style, noted psychiatrist Dr. Helen DeRosis will show women of today how to manage anxiety in an easy step-by-step program. With sensible suggestions and solutions, this book will show you how to turn anxiety into a positive force in your life and how to learn to channel it in healthy and constructive ways.

'A book every woman-married, single, working, or home-oriented-could use
to help her live a fuller, free-of-fear life."
— *Ladies Home Journal*

"a timely, well-written guide that ought to go a long way in helping today
women cope with the stresses of modem life. "
— *San Francisco Sunday Examiner & Chronicle*

Dr. Helen A. DeRosis is a practicing psychiatrist who has devoted years of study and research of the mental health problems of women. Associate Clinical Professor in Psychiatry at New York University School of Medicine, Dr. DeRosis has been a frequent guest on many national television shows, including *Donohue!*, *Good Morning America* and *Today*. A native New Yorker, Dr. DeRosis is also the author of the bestsellers *The Book of Hope* and *Parent Power/Child Power*. She is currently organizing a pilot, grass-roots, family-aid program in the South Bronx, *Parents for the Prevention of Violence*.

PRICE	PAGES	ISBN	CATEGORY
$14.95 Pbk.	272	1-886330-99-9	Women Studies/Self-help

Available at bookstores everywhere or direct from the publisher at
1-800-906-1234.
Visit our health and self-help website www.takecommand.com

RESILIENCE:
How to Bounce Back When the Going Gets Tough!
by Frederic Flach, M.D.

THERE'S no escaping stress. It appears on our doorstep uninvited in the shattering forms of death and divorce, or even in the pleasant experiences of promotion, marriage, or a long-held wish fulfilled. Anything that upsets the delicate balance of our daily lives creates stress. So why do some people come out of acrisis feeling better than ever, and others never seem quite themselves again?

Drawing on thirty years of case studies from his own psychiatric practice, Dr. Flach reveals the remarkable antidote to the destructive qualities of stress: RESILIENCE.

Readers will discover:

• How to develop the 14 traits that will make you more resilient
• Why "falling apart" is the smartest step to take on the road to resilience
• How to break down your body's resilience blockers and gain strength
• The sanity-saving technique of distracting yourself
• The helpful five-step plan for creative problem solving
• How developing your self-worth and your own unique gifts leads to resilience
• The power of language to destroy and to heal
• How to redefine your problem and restructure your pain to create a life you can handle, a life you can learn from and enjoy!

> "Part practical and part inspirational .... Written with clarity.. contains short, readable examples for all aspects of life ... useful to laypersons in times of crisis. "
>
> *—The New England Journal of Medicine*

Frederic Flach, MD., is an intentionally recognized psychiatrist and author, who has devoted more than thirty years of practice, scientific research, and teaching in the development of his own personal perspective of resilience. Dr. Each graduated from Cornell University Medical College, where he currently serves as Adjunct Associate Professor of Psychiatry and is Attending Psychiatrist at both the Payne Whitney Clinic of the New York Hospital and St. Vincent's Hospital and Medical Center. In addition to numerous articles in scientific journals, he is also the author of the bestseller, *The Secret Strength of Depression* (1995), *Putting the Pieces Together Again* (1996).

PRICE	PAGES	ISBN	CATEGORY
$14.95 Pbk	270	1-886330-95-6	Self-help/Psychology

Available at bookstores everywhere or direct from the publisher at
1-800-906-1234.
Visit our health and self-help website www.takecommand.com

CLIMB A FALLEN LADDER
How to Survive (and Thrive!) in a Downsized America
by Rochelle H. Gordon, MD and Catherine E. Harold
Foreword by Ron P. Simmons, co-author of the bestseller
Value-Directed Management

"Can I see you in my office please?"

LATE on a Friday afternoon, those are the last words you want to hear from the Human Resources Manager or your supervisor. That knot in your stomach says you're about to join the millions of your fellow Americans who have been downsized, re-engineered, or restructured after years of loyal employment.

Now there's hope and guidance for the millions of people who have been downsized, the "working worried" still clinging to long-held jobs, their families, and their friends, in *Climb a Fallen Ladder*.

Dr. Rochelle Gordon and Catherine Harold offer inspiring and instructive stories of real people and proven principles for coping and thriving in this new age of anxiety. Although everyone is talking about downsizing, no one is talking to the workers. *Climb a Fallen Ladder* is the first book about downsizing to address employees' emotional and psychological needs. It will help displaced or despairing workers cope with the crisis, maintain dignity and a sense of self at work and at home, and take command of life at the most vulnerable time.

Destined to become a classic, *Climb a Fallen Ladder* is for everyone who works or wants to.

With very special sections on:

• The Working Worried: How To Stay Stable When Your Job Isn't

• Getting Laid Off: What to Expect and How To Thrive!

• Family Matters: In Troubled Times Call On the Troops

Rochelle H. Gordon is the first woman ever to chair the psychiatry department at the John Muir Medical Center in Walnut Creek, California. A native New Yorker, Dr. Gordon has had a private practice in the San Francisco Bay Area for over twenty years. Dr. Gordon specializes in the treatment of professionals and executives coping with corporate reorganization and job anxiety

Catherine E Harold was recently downsized herself from a large healthcare conglomerate. A professional writer and editor for more than 15 years, Ms. Harold has edited more than 30 books and written scores of magazine article on health related topics. She resides in Tucson, Arizona.

PRICE	PAGES	ISBN	CATEGORY
$21.95 hc	250	1-886330-96-4	Business/Self-help

Available at bookstores everywhere or direct from the publisher at
1-800-906-1234.
Visit our health and self-help website www.takecommand.com

PUTTING THE PIECES TOGETHER AGAIN

by Frederic Flach, MD

E VERY once in a while, readers discover a special book that has tremendous potential to change the way they live their lives. Call it wisdom — or perhaps the knowledge to develop a personal philosophy — presented in a subtle yet powerful way, *Putting the Pieces Together Again* is such a book.

Putting the Pieces Together Again was first published in 1976. The idea that we all have a right, in fact a need, to fall apart sometimes when faced with stress or change strongly captured the minds and hearts of innumerable readers.

Before Dr. Flach wrote this book, the idea that falling apart-being temporarily immobilized by stress, for example-could serve any helpful purpose was alien to our way of thinking. Dr. Flach shows how "falling apart" can often be the only healthy response to stress setting the stage for major advances in psychological growth.

Putting the Pieces Together Again is a stimulating and inspiring look at stress, creativity and change. Today, more than ever, "readers have much to gain from the wisdom and insight offered in this book"

—Library Journal

Dr. Flach is Adjunct Associate Professor of psychiatry at Cornell University Medical College and Attending Psychiatrist at both The New York Hospital-Cornell Medical Center and Saint Vincent's Hospital and Medical Center of New York. His clinical interests have focused on the subjects of depression and stress management for 30 years. His books have included *A New Marriage, A New Life* and the bestsellers *Resilience* and *Rickie*. He has been a guest on many national television broadcasts, including *Good Morning America, The Today Show, Sally Jesse Raphael,* and *Donahue!*

PRICE	PAGES	ISBN	CATEGORY
$8.95 Ppb.	212	1-886330-03-4	Psychology/Self-help

Available at bookstores everywhere or direct from the publisher at 1-800-906-1234.
Visit our health and self-help website www.takecommand.com

STOP WORRYING ABOUT MONEY!
How to Take Control of Your Financial Life

by Mitch "The Money Buddy" Gallon

A simple and easy-to-understand guide for managing your money

EVERYONE worries about money and fear of finances prevents millions of people from addressing their money woes — leading to overwhelming debt and inability to save money. *Stop Worrying About Money!* provides an innovative, step-by-step program designed to take the fear and mystery out of managing your money. It will help you feel more confident about yourself and teach you to handle your personal finances without fear or pain.

Stop Worrying About Money! will show you how to:

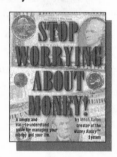

- Stop buying on impulse
- Set aside a nest egg for a rainy day or even a sunny day
- Perform plastic surgery on those credit card bills
- Set realistic financial goals...and stick to them
- Reduce stress and feel good about yourself

Mitch "The Money Buddy" Gallon is a professional bookkeeper with over 18 years of experience. Her other accomplishments include registered nursing, nightclub promotion, and house building. She is the creator of the famous Money Buddy Personal Wealth Management System and the founder of the Benebook Library Fund, which distributes books to inner city libraries. A native of Baltimore, a wife and mother, she now resides in Ellicott City Maryland.

PRICE	PAGES	ISBN	CATEGORY
$11.95 Pbk.	168	1-886330-93-X	Personal Finance/Self-help

Available at bookstores everywhere or direct from the publisher at
1-800-906-1234.
Visit our health and self-help website www.takecommand.com